Techniques of Botulinum Toxin Injections in the Head and Neck

Techniques of Botulinum Toxin Injections in the Head and Neck

Michael S. Benninger, MD
P. Daniel Knott, MD

PLURAL PUBLISHING
INC.
SAN DIEGO
OXFORD
MELBOURNE

PLURAL PUBLISHING
INC.

5521 Ruffin Road
San Diego, CA 92123

e-mail: info@pluralpublishing.com
Web site: http://www.pluralpublishing.com

49 Bath Street
Abingdon, Oxfordshire OX14 1EA
United Kingdom

Typeset in 10.5/13 Palatino Book by Flanagan's Publishing Services, Inc.
Printed in the United States of America by Bang Printing

Benninger, Michael S.
Techniques of botulinum toxin injections in the head and neck / Michael S. Benninger and P. Daniel Knott.
p. ; cm.
Includes bibliographical references and index.
ISBN-13: 978-1-59756-442-7 (alk. paper)
ISBN-10: 1-59756-442-7 (alk. paper)
I. Knott, P. Daniel (Philip Daniel) II. Title.
[DNLM: 1. Botulinum Toxins—therapeutic use. 2. Dystonia—drug therapy. 3. Head. 4. Neck. 5. Synkinesis—drug therapy. QV 140]
LC Classification not assigned
615.9'5—dc23
2012011987

Contents

Foreword by Gayle Woodson

George Bernard Shaw once said "All great truths begin as blasphemies." When I first heard the suggestion that botulinum toxin might be used to treat spasmodic dysphonia (SD), I dismissed the thought as incredible. How could the use of such a potent lethal neurotoxin possibly be justified for treatment of a benign (albeit disabling) condition? However, I also had misgivings about the variability of outcomes for spasmodic dysphonia patients after recurrent laryngeal nerve section. My colleague at Baylor Medical School, Joe Jancovic, was effectively managing other dystonias with botulinum toxin, and some of his patients sounded just like my SD patients! And so Robert Miller and I collaborated with Jancovic in using the toxin to treat patients with SD. Our initial idea was that we could use botulinum toxin to select patients for recurrent laryngeal nerve transection. The toxin could provide a trial of paralysis that would be significantly longer than that produced by injection of lidocaine. We began by injecting 30 units into one vocal fold. We did not know what to expect, and so we admitted the first patient to the ICU for observation after the injection. Rather anticlimactically, the only ill effect was a mildly breathy voice. The vocal fold, though weak, was not paralyzed, and we concluded that paralysis was not necessary to improve speech. And thus, the potent lethal neurotoxin became a very attractive alternative treatment for patients with SD.

In 1989, the Food and Drug Administration (FDA) approved botulinum toxin for treatment of strabismus, blepharospasm, and hemifacial spasm. The following year, the National Institutes of Health (NIH) convened a Consensus Conference on the Clinical Uses of Botulinum Toxin, and we presented our experience with SD. I was amazed that the toxin was useful in such a wide variety of conditions. The cost of conducting studies to support FDA approval for every single indication of the toxin would be staggering; the 1990 NIH conference collated and validated the necessary literature to support non-FDA approved uses.

I thought it was heresy when I first heard that botulinum toxin was effective in treating wrinkles. My colleague at UCSD at the time, Michael Swenson, joked that we could establish an "Institute of Cosmetic Toxicology." But the cosmetic applications have ultimately eclipsed the medical indications for the toxin. In popular culture, botulinum toxin is now regarded as a vanity drug, and we have to keep this medication locked up to prevent pilfering. It is therefore very heartening to see this book, dedicated to the full spectrum of the clinical applications of this amazing substance. The ultimate message of botulinum toxin is the importance of keeping an open mind—because who knows what seemingly outlandish ideas could ultimately lead to better treatment for our patients.

Gayle Woodson, MD
Professor and Chair of Otolaryngology
Southern Illinois University School of Medicine
Springfield, Illinois

Foreword by Corey S. Maas

Drs. Benninger and Knott have provided the clinician a useful reference guide for applications of botulinum toxins in the head and neck region. Their efforts are particularly utilitarian as they effectively cover both the functional and aesthetic applications of this powerful tool and its primary applications—the head and neck.

As otolaryngologists and facial plastic surgeons are uniquely qualified to apply the techniques described in *Techniques of Botulinum Toxin Injections in the Head and Neck*, this simple, well-referenced guide is a perfect addition as a desktop reference.

The authors provide unit dosages for both Botox (Botox Cosmetic) and Dysport, with comprehensive lists of conditions in which these products are indicated. In reviewing these dosage recommendations, they are in the conservative range relative to consensus publications and thus provide safety margins for those starting to use these products, as well as an excellent starting point for experienced clinicians who are seeking to expand their indications.

This field changes very quickly; Xeomin has recently been introduced to the market, and is well-established in Germany as a Botox alternative. My early experience with Xeomin suggests, in contradistinction to some published reports, that dose ratios of Botox to Xeomin are not 1:1 but closer to 1:1.2. Xeomin and Purtox (Mentor Corp, Santa Barbara, CA), which is in late-stage clinical trials, together with those products discussed in *Techniques of Botulinum Toxin Injections in the Head and Neck*, may dramatically change the landscape of the "pharma world" from that of Botox to a more physician-controlled commoditization of the neuromodulators or, more precisely, myomodulators.

Drs. Benninger and Knott are to be commended for their fine work in keeping the information concise, clinically oriented, and indication-specific. This book should be on the desktop of all who use myomodulators.

Corey S. Maas, MD, FACS
Associate Clinical Professor
University of California, San Francisco
San Francisco, California

Preface

Since the introduction of botulinum toxin for injections in humans initially for dystonias such as blephorospasm, the unique characteristics of the drug have led to adaptation of botulinum toxin for use in multiple medical indications. These range from dystonias to muscle contraction disorders, pain disorders, and cosmetics. Although many of the uses are throughout the body, a majority of indications for use are within the head and neck region. Some of these are related to initial use in various head and neck dystonias, although newer applications seem to be identified each year. Not only are there more and more applications, there appears to be some variability of techniques within some disorders and variability in dosing. The evolution to newer types of botulinum toxin also raises confusion as to equivalency of dosing.

This book aims to create a simple, directed reference showing the specific techniques of performing botulinum toxin injections in the head and neck. It is not meant as an overarching reference on botulinum toxin use nor an in-depth discussion of the various conditions for which it has been applied. Chapter 1 discusses the development and history of botulinum toxin in medicine, its action, and the relative differences between its various types. The remainder of the book serves as a technical atlas, describing the specific techniques for injection and the possible dosing levels for a variety of head and neck conditions. These techniques are well illustrated to allow for use as a quick technical reference. The pertinent anatomic muscle groups are presented in each chapter, with illustrations.

The techniques illustrated here may not represent all approaches to various conditions but are a synopsis of the most common approaches described in the literature and recommendations based on the authors' experiences. As there are a variety of types of botulinum toxin and products produced by more than one manufacturer, the term botulinum toxin is used to describe a generic toxin, although it applies almost exclusively to botulinum toxin type A. When the authors use specific terms, such as Botox or Dysport, they are referring to specific products. These are largely determined by our preference and experience and do not refute the use of other products. All techniques described only identify doses for botulinum type A, although an approximate equivalency chart is noted in Chapter 1. Although the Food and Drug Administration (FDA) has approved Botox for injection in humans and for specific indications, not all injection techniques discussed are specifically FDA approved.

We hope you enjoy the simplicity of the techniques described, so that it can serve as a quick and helpful reference in everyday practice.

Acknowledgment

The authors would like to acknowledge the efforts and patience of Beth Halasz in illustrating this book. A work of this kind is particularly dependent upon accurate, simplified, yet beautiful figures. Ms. Halasz, in spite of considerable pressure to dedicate her time and attention to other projects, laboriously researched, completed, and endlessly revised each illustration. We are deeply in debt to Ms. Halasz's grace, professionalism, and artistry.

Contributing Authors

Michael S. Benninger, MD
Chairman, Head and Neck Institute
The Cleveland Clinic
Cleveland, Ohio
Sections I and II Introductions, and Chapters 2 through 9

Anne F. Hseu, MD
Head and Neck Institute
The Cleveland Clinic
Cleveland, Ohio
Chapter 1

Andrea Jarchow, MD
Assistant Professor
Division of Facial Plastic and Reconstructive Surgery
Department of Otolaryngology-Head and Neck Surgery
University of North Carolina–Chapel Hill
Chapel Hill, North Carolina
Chapter 14

P. Daniel Knott, MD, FACS
Associate Professor
Director, Facial Plastic and Reconstructive Surgery
Department of Otolaryngology—Head and Neck Surgery
University of California, San Francisco
San Francisco, California
Section III Introduction, and Chapters 11, 12, 13, 15, and 16

Peter C. Revenaugh, MD
Head and Neck Institute
The Cleveland Clinic
Cleveland, Ohio
Chapter 10

CHAPTER

1

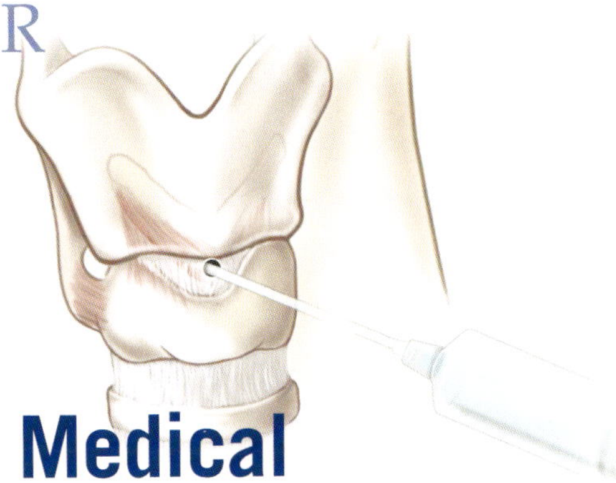

Botox in Medical Applications: History, Types of Toxin, and Doses

Anne F. Hseu

INTRODUCTION

Botulinum toxin is a medication and neurotoxic protein produced by the bacterium *Clostridium botulinum*. The bacterium is a gram-positive, obligate anaerobic bacillus that produces spores. These spores can be found in vegetables, fruits, and seafood, whereas *C. botulinum* is found in soil and marine sediment.[1] Poisoning by the bacterium results in symptoms of autonomic dysfunction, which may include dry mouth or postural hypotension. Victims can exhibit muscle paralysis potentially leading to suffocation and death.

Once a poison, botulinum toxin is currently one of the most versatile medications in the treatment of human disorders. Applications are vast across specialties such as ophthalmology, otolaryngology, dermatology, and neurology. Although *C. botulinum* and its toxins have been studied for hundreds of years, research into its mechanisms of action and future medical applications continues to this day.

HISTORICAL CONTEXT

Although food-borne botulism likely has been present since ancient times, there are few historical sources and documents on its toxicity prior to the 18th and 19th centuries.[2] Early dietary taboos and food edicts, however, may have reflected some knowledge of the existence of botulism poisoning. For instance, in the 10th century, Emperor Leo VI of Byzantium (886–911) forbade the manufacturing of blood sausages.[3] Some reported cases of belladonna toxicity at the time, in fact, may have also been due to botulism as dilated pupils and muscle paralysis alone cannot be attributed to atropine intoxication.[2]

In the 18th and 19th centuries, multiple cases of fatal food poisoning were noted in the southwest region of Wurttemberg, Germany. Economic poverty caused by the Napoleonic wars (1795–1813) had decreased hygiene standards for food production in the rural areas. In 1793, a severe outbreak of food poisoning occurred in the small village of Wildbad where 6 persons died.[2] It was speculated that victims' fatal muscle paralysis was related to the consumption of smoked blood sausages. As such, the word botulism stems from the Greek word for sausage, *botulus*.

The first publications on "sausage poisoning" are credited to Justinus Kerner, a German poet and medical officer who lived in the small town of Welzheim.[4] He is noted to be the first person to accurately describe the symptoms of food-borne botulism and suggest its potential therapeutic use. Kerner's first monograph, published in 1820, was entitled, "New Observations on the Lethal Poisoning Occurring So Frequently in Wurttemberg Through the Consumption of Smoked Sausages." In this monograph, Kerner detailed 76 cases of botulinum toxicity and accurately described its symptoms, time course, and physical findings. His second monograph, "The Fat Poison or the Fatty Acid and Its Effects on the Animal Organism, a Contribution to the Substance Which Acts Toxically in Bad Sausages," postulated that the botulinum toxin acted by interrupting transmission of the peripheral and autonomic nervous system.

Although Kerner made great strides in the description of botulism, it was not until 1895 that microbiologist Emile Van Ermengem identified bacteria as the causative agent in the food poisoning. Van Ermengem had been appointed to investigate a fatal outbreak of botulism that occurred in the Belgian village of Ellezelles on December 14, 1895. On that fateful day, 34 people had gathered to eat at the wake of 87-year-old Antoine Creteur. After a meal of smoked ham, multiple persons were noted to have symptoms of dry mouth, ileus, hypotension, and flaccid paralysis. According to reports, 23 people were paralyzed and 3 people died.[2] Through detailed examinations of the food and its victims, Van Ermengem was able to isolate a causative anaerobic organism, which he called *Bacillus botulinus*. The name was later changed to *Clostridium botulinum* but not before Van Ermengem published his findings in 1897.

Thirty-one years later in 1928, Dr. Herman Sommer and colleagues at UCSF were able to purify botulinum toxin as a stable acid precipitate.[5] This proved invaluable, as the world had turned its attention toward chemical and biological warfare. In fact, during World War II (1939–1945), foreign intelligence reports in the United States had indicated that many countries were engaged in biowarfare programs. Therefore, in response, the U.S. Academy of Sciences set up a laboratory named Fort Detrick in Maryland for offensive and defensive biowarfare research.[6]

Although botulinum toxin is the most poisonous substance known to man, it is no longer considered an ideal weapon. A single gram evenly dispersed and inhaled has the capacity to kill more than one million people.[6] However, several factors limit its use as a biological weapon. First, in order to be lethal, botulinum toxin must be ingested in sufficient quantities. Even then, mortality rates with ingestion are variable. Second, the toxin is rapidly inactivated by standard water sanitation protocols. Third, it is not transmissible from one person to another. Finally, botulinum toxicity can be effectively treated with antitoxin or broad-spectrum antibiotics.[7] In fact, during World War II, there were concerns that Germany had weaponized the toxin, therefore toxoid vaccines were prepared for Allied troops prior to the invasion of Normandy on D-Day.[6]

Nonetheless, researchers at Fort Detrick were able to make great strides in botulinum research. In 1946, Dr. Edward Schantz first purified the neurotoxin for use in humans. Although President Nixon ordered Fort Detrick closed in 1972 after the Biological and Toxins Weapons Convention Treaty was signed, Schantz continued his research at the University of Wisconsin. There, he was able to manufacture toxin in a concentrated form for experimental use and provided the product to the academic community.[4]

MEDICINAL USE

In the early 1970s, ophthalmologist Dr. Alan Scott began investigating the use of botulinum toxin in animals as a potential treatment for strabismus.[8] Because strabismus had such high reoperation rates, other alternatives to surgical treatment were being sought. This included injectable anesthetics, enzymes, alcohol, and enzyme blockers, as well as various neurotoxins.[4] Scott found botulinum A exotoxin to be the most effective, as a few picograms induced long-lasting paralysis that remained confined to the injected muscle. In addition to this, no apparent side effects were seen.[4] The result of Scott's animal studies were published in 1973 and subsequently, an application for human use was submitted to the U.S. Food and Drug Administration (FDA).[9] Clinical trials in humans began in 1977. By 1982, ophthalmologists were injecting botulinum toxin for strabismus, nystagmus, lid retraction, hemifacial spasm, and blepharospasm. Other physicians were injecting limbs and the neck for dystonia. The results of Scott's large multicenter trial were published in 1989; the publication documented approximately 17,000 treatment sessions in over 7,000 patients.[10] The same year, the FDA approved the use of botulinum toxin in strabismus, blepharospasm, and hemifacial spasm. FDA approval for other indications followed shortly thereafter.

MECHANISM OF ACTION

Clostridium botulinum is a phylogenetically heterogeneous species, categorized as consisting of seven different serotypes. Each produces an antigenically distinct toxin, designated A through G. The serotypes all have similar weights and structure and efficacy but they differ in their target proteins.[11] Currently, only types A and B have clinical application.

Regardless of serotype, botulinum toxin consists of a heavy chain of 100 kDa and a light chain of 50 kDa, which are bridged by a disulfide bond. The heavy chain is responsible for selectively and irreversibly binding the neurotoxin to receptors on the surface of presynaptic cholinergic cells. Consequently, the toxin is endocytosed and the disulfide bond is cleaved as the pH in the vesicle decreases. The light chain then functions as an endopeptidase to disrupt proteins necessary for the exocytosis of acetylcholine-containing vesicles. This causes an irreversible blockade of cholinergic transmission at ganglionic synapses, postganglionic parasympathetic synapses, and neuromuscular junctions.[12]

The complex of proteins targeted by the toxin is called the SNARE complex. This family of proteins normally facilitates the docking of neurotransmitter vesicles to the presynaptic membrane. Each botulinum toxin serotype has specific molecular targets in the SNARE complex. For instance, type A cleaves 9 amino acids from the C-terminal of SNAP-25 and type B cleaves vesicle-associated membrane protein (VAMP).[13]

Recovery from botulinum toxin involves two phases. During the first phase, new axons appear and allow for limited acetylcholine release. In the second phase, new synthesis of the SNARE complex proteins occurs.[14] After a little more than 90 days, recovery is essentially complete. This is why patients require repeat injections every few months to maintain a sustained effect. However, duration of neurotransmitter inhibition does vary according to serotype. Type A is of the longest duration; type B is slightly shorter (Table 1–1).

Table 1–1. *Types of Botulinum Toxin*

Types	Protein Targets[11]	Brand Names	Duration of Paralysis[15,16]
A	SNAP-25	Botox, Dysport, Neuronox, Xeomin, Reloxin, Azzalure	4–6 months
B	VAMP/ Synaptobrevin	Myobloc, Neurobloc	3 months
C	SNAP-25 & Syntaxin		4–5 months
D	VAMP/ Synaptobrevin		Human neurons lack specific receptor[13]
E	SNAP-25		1 month
F	VAMP/ Synaptobrevin		2 months

DOSAGE AND TOXICITY

At present, absolute contraindications to use of botulinum toxin include pregnancy and breast-feeding because its effect is unknown. Relative contraindications include preexisting neuromuscular conditions and drug use, which might potentiate the effect of the toxin.

Botulinum toxin is relatively well tolerated but there can be complications and adverse reactions. Most commonly, diffusion to a nearby muscle can occur, causing unintentional weakening. There are also case reports of generalized weakness and reactions, which are postulated to be related to small amounts of toxin diffusion into the circulation.[11] Side effects can include injection site reactions. Long-term use may cause denervation atrophy, although sometimes this is the therapeutic goal.

Although it was first discovered as a poison, there have been no reported deaths secondary to overdose in over 35 years of human use. The estimated lethal dose of a 70 kg person is 2800 U, which is far higher than dosages normally used.

COMMERCIAL USAGE

At present, there are two well-known commercial preparations of botulinum toxin type A: Botox and Dysport. Botox is more commonly used in the United States, whereas Dysport is used more commonly in Europe. Manufactured by Allergan, Botox is nearly 4 times more effective than Dysport in similar doses. Botox, therefore, is available in 100-unit vials whereas Dysport is sold in 500-unit vials.

One of the primary complications of botulinum toxin therapy has been the formation of antibodies to type-A toxin. This obliterates treatment response, therefore other serotypes have been sought for therapeutic use. Unfortunately, none of the other serotypes appear to have the potency or duration of action of type A.[17] Type B botulinum, however, has been manufactured under the name Myobloc. Although type B is more often associated with autonomic side effects, its production has become invaluable for patients that develop antibodies to type A.

Currently, botulinum toxin is manufactured in a crystalline form and is diluted with normal saline. The recommendation is to use the reconstituted toxin within 4 hours but this recommendation is currently being studied and challenged.

REFERENCES

1. Lamanna C. The most poisonous poison. *Science.* 1959 Sep 25;130: 763–772.
2. Erbguth FJ. Historical notes on botulism, Clostridium botulinum, botulinum toxin, and the idea of the therapeutic use of the toxin. *Mov Disord.* 2004 Mar;19 (suppl 8):S2–6.
3. Smith L. *Botulism. The Organism, Its Toxins, the Disease.* Springfield IL: Charles C. Thomas Publishers; 1977.
4. Scott AB. Development of botulinum toxin therapy. *Dermatol Clin.* 2004 Apr;22(2):131–133.
5. Snipe PT, Sommer H. Studies on botulinus toxin: 3. Acid precipitation of botulinus toxin. *J Infect Dis.* 1928 Aug:43(2):152–160.
6. Arnon SS, Schechter R, Inglesby TV, et al. Botulinum toxin as a biological weapon: medical and public health management. *JAMA.* 2001 Feb 28;285(8):1059–1070.
7. Ting PT, Freiman A. The story of Clostridium botulinum: from food poisoning to Botox. *Clin Med.* 2004 May–June;4(3):258–261.
8. Carruthers A, Carruthers J. History of the cosmetic use of botulinum A exotoxin. *Dermatol Surg.* 1998 Nov;24(11):1168–1170.
9. Scott AB, Rosenbaum A, Collins CC. Pharmacologic weakening of extraocular muscles. *Invest Ophthalmol.* 1973;12:924–927.
10. Scott AB. In: Simpson LL, ed. *Clostridial Toxins as Therapeutic Agents in Botulinum Neurotoxin and Tetanus Toxin.* Academic Press: 1989; 399–409.
11. Aoki KR, Guyer B. Botulinum toxin type A and other botulinum toxin serotypes: a comparative review of biochemical and pharmacological actions. *Eur J Neurol.* 2001 Nov;8 (suppl 5):21–29.

12. Caya JG, Agni R, Miller JE. Clostridium botulinum and the clinical laboratorian: a detailed review of botulism, including biological warfare ramifications of botulinum toxin. *Arch Pathol Lab Med.* 2004 June;128(6):653–662.
13. Davletov B, Bajohrs M, Binz T. Beyond BOTOX: advantages and limitations of individual botulinum neurotoxins. *Trends Neurosci.* 2005 Aug;28(8):446–452.
14. Wenzel RG. Pharmacology of botulinum neurotoxin serotype A. *Am J Health Syst Pharm.* 2004 Nov 15;61(22 suppl 6):S5–10.
15. Foran PG, Davletov B, Meunier FA. Getting muscles moving again after botulinum toxin: novel therapeutic challenges. *Trends Mol Med.* 2003;9:291–299.
16. Meunier FA, Lisk G, Sesardic D, Dolly JO. Dynamics of motor nerve terminal remodeling unveiled using SNARE-cleaving botulinum toxins: the extent and duration are dictated by the sites of SNAP-25 truncation. *Mol Cell Neurosci.* 2003 Apr;22(4):454–466.
17. Johnson EA. Clostridial toxins as therapeutic agents: benefits of nature's most toxic proteins. *Annu Rev Microbiol.* 1999;53:551–575.

SECTION

I

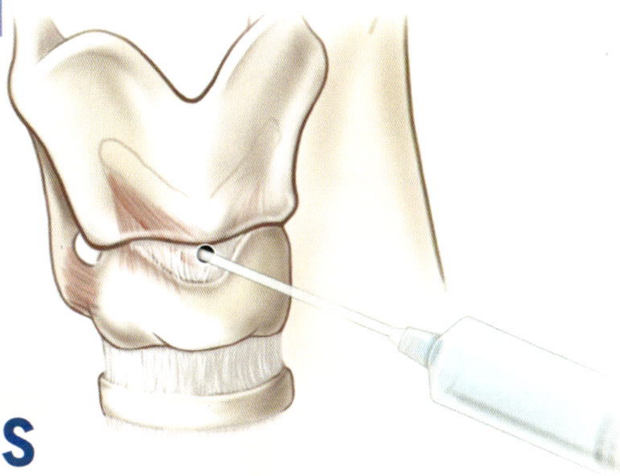

Dystonias

Michael S. Benninger

Dystonia is a term that describes an abnormal muscle movement characterized by repetitive involuntary muscle contractions. It is thought to be a neurological condition and the various contractions are described as sustained (tonic) or spasmodic (clonic). Depending on the size and location of the muscle contractions there can be gross posturing and disfigurement during the activity, although the muscle action is usually normal during rest. Typically, these dystonic contractions are induced by conscious action to move the muscle group.[1,2] Dystonia can be categorized based on the amount of muscle involvement as generalized, segmental, or focal. Generalized dystonias describes widespread muscle activity whereas focal dystonias involve only one or a few local small muscles. Segmental dystonias are abnormal muscle contraction of neighboring groups of muscles.[3]

There has been much debate and investigation as to the etiology of dystonias and often there is a precipitating event such as trauma or infection. Some of the dystonias have strong family inheritance patterns although most are sporadic. There has been an association with various other neurological diseases such as other muscle group dystonias and tremor, and disorders such as neurological injury or insults, neurodegenerative disorders, and tardive syndromes.[1] Most dystonias, however, are idiopathic. Because of the relationship with a number of other neurologic diseases or other dystonias a neurologic evaluation and recommendation for potential medical therapies should be considered. There are multiple potential treatments for the muscle contractions of the various dystonias including medications, and physical, occupational, or voice therapy. One of the principal treatments is the use of botulinum toxin to block the muscular contractions. Botulinum toxin has both the advantage of few side effects and predictable results in many conditions, although patients almost always require repeat injection.

REFERENCES

1. Cultrara A, Chitkara A, Blitzer A. Botulinum toxin injections for the treatment of oromandibular dystonia. *Oper Tech Otolaryngol Head Neck Surg*. 2004;15:97–102.
2. Fahn S. The varied clinical expressions of dystonia. *Neurol Clin*. 1984;2:541–554.
3. Fahn S. Concept and classification of dystonia. *Adv Neurol*. 1988;50:1–8.

CHAPTER

2

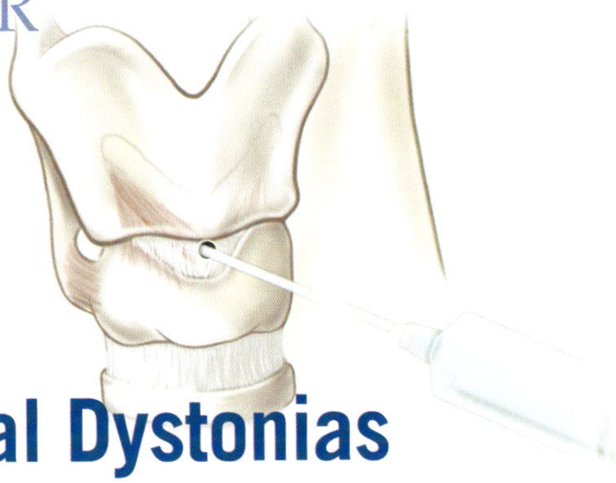

Laryngeal Dystonias

Michael S. Benninger

Although there are a number of laryngeal dystonias, the most commonly encountered laryngeal dystonia is spasmodic dysphonia (SD). Spasmodic dysphonia is a focal dystonia of the larynx. It is subdivided into an adductor type (adductor SD) where the vocal folds spasm in adduction and an abductor type (abductor SD) where the vocal folds spasm or contract in abduction. Adductor SD accounts for 80 to 90% of all cases and abductor SD accounts for between 10 to 20%.[1] There are a small group of patients who have both and abductor and adductor component (<1%) and the treatment of such patients can be particularly challenging.

Patients with adductor SD have pitch breaks, irregular speech, and a strained or strangled voice whereas individuals with abductor SD have a breathy quality to the voice with a short duration of vocalization due to excessive air loss on phonation. This is particularly true in words that begin with a voiceless consonant followed by a vowel (such as pat or puppy). The primary treatment for SD is with Botox injections with a very high initial and subsequent success rate in treating adductor SD.[2] With abductor SD, responses are more variable with Botox injections.[1]

ANATOMIC CONSIDERATIONS

The two primary muscles that are injected for SD are the thyroarytenoid muscle (vocalis muscle) and the posterior cricoarytenoid muscle. The thyroarytenoid muscle is a primary tensor of the vocal fold and has a medial and a lateral belly that blend into one muscle group. Although they have slightly different effects on tensing the vocal folds, these differences are minor and do not seem to have an impact on the effectiveness of the botulinum toxin injections. The muscle attaches anteriorly to the thyroid cartilage via Broyle's ligament in the area of the macula flava. When seen anteriorly, the insertion is usually in the midpoint of the distance between the thyroid notch and the lower boarder of the thyroid cartilage. The medial belly of the muscle inserts posteriorly to the muscular process of the arytenoid cartilage medially and the lateral belly attaches to the body of the arytenoid more laterally.[3]

The posterior cricoarytenoid muscle is the only true abductor of the vocal folds, although the cricothyroid muscle may have some abductor role in deep inspiration. It opens the glottis by separating the vocal folds by rotating the arytenoid cartilage laterally and tilting it. There are paired muscles on each side. The posterior cricoarytenoid muscle is a broad muscle with its origin along a broad depression on the posterior surface of the posterior lamina of the cricoid cartilage. The muscle fibers then converge and insert on the muscular process of the arytenoid.[3]

TECHNIQUES FOR ADDUCTOR SD

There are a number of approaches to the injection of Botox for adductor SD. The most common approach is through the cricothyroid membrane, but the injections can also be made through the thyrohyoid membrane or from above through the mouth either with a long curved needle or through a flexible endoscope. Injections can also be made into both or one vocal fold. The typical starting dose for bilateral vocal fold injections is 2.0 or 2.5 units a side into the thyroarytenoid muscle. The patients may note a period of breathiness beginning a day or 2 after the injection and this may last from 1 to 2 days to a couple of weeks. During that time, the patient may be more susceptible to aspiration when ingesting thin liquids and should do so cautiously if they are very breathy. Although the length of the effect may be variable typical results will last between 3 to 6 months. Over the last month or so the individual will note gradually increasing strain and effort.

The amount of Botox injected on subsequent visits will depend on a number of factors including the degree and length of postinjection breathiness and the length of time between the injection and the return of symptoms. The dose is tempered by the desire of the patient. Some individuals cannot tolerate much breathiness but are willing to accept more frequent injections, in which case the starting dose will be decreased on subsequent injections, whereas others may not care about the breathiness but may want a more sustained effect and less frequent injections. In this case the dose can be left as is or increased. There are unique individuals who continue to have significant periods of breathiness after injections of even small amounts of Botox. In these cases, an option is to do a higher dose of Botox injected into one vocal fold. An approximate equivalency between the dose of Botox in one vocal fold in comparison to both vocal folds varies slightly as the dose increases (Table 2–1).[4]

Injection Through the Cricothyroid Membrane

This injection can be performed either with EMG localization or observing the vocal folds from above with a flexible scope.

Table 2–1. *Equivalency Doses for Unilateral in Comparison to Bilateral Vocal Fold Injections for Spasmodic Dysphonia*[4]

Unilateral	Bilateral
1.25–2.5 units	No equivalence
5 units	0.625 units
10–15 units	1.25 units
25–30 units	2.5 units

In many cases it is simpler and quicker to use EMG localization. The injection can be performed in either a sitting or supine position. A small amount of xylocaine can be injected into the cricothyroid space and then into the tracheal lumen (Fig 2–1). A hollow-bore elctromyographic needle is passed through the cricothyroid space, and directed superiorly and laterally into the vocal fold until muscle motor potentials are identified. Position is confirmed by seeing an increase in motor unit potentials and the Botox is injected. The needle can then be directed superiorly and laterally into the other vocal fold without withdrawing the needle from the neck. The entire procedure typically can be performed in less than a minute or two. A similar technique can be used for the treatment of primary vocal tremor although the results are more variable.

Injections Through the Thyrohyoid Space

Similar to the technique above, this can be performed either with EMG guidance or with direct visualization above with a flexible scope, although the angles make it simpler to use a flexible endoscope to visualize the needle. Local anesthesia can be performed by injection into the skin just above the

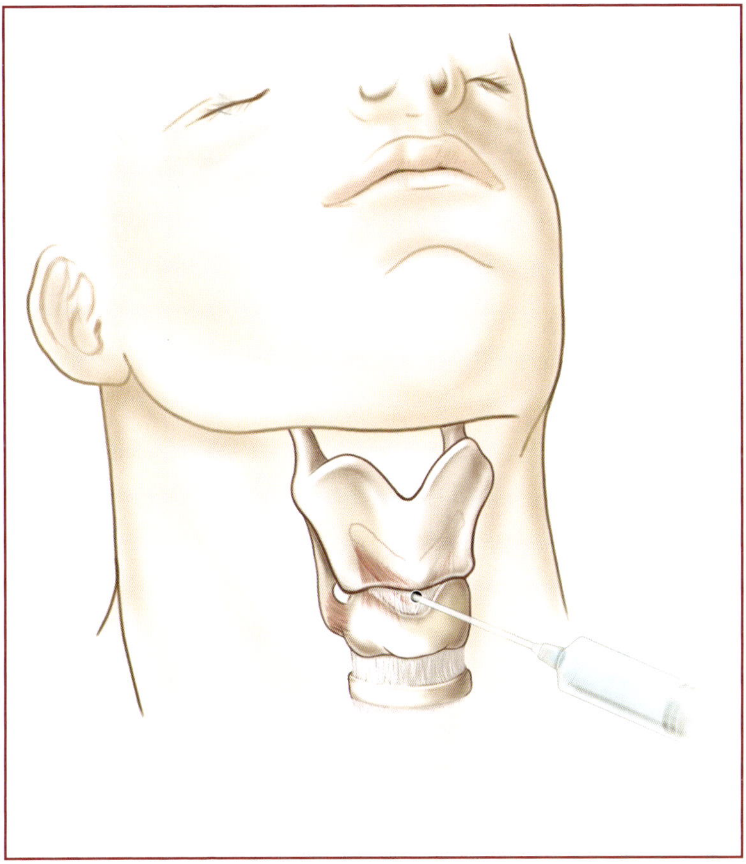

Figure 2–1

thyroid notch and into the deeper tissues. The needle is then passed in the midline just above the thyroid notch, directed inferiorly, and visualized as it enters into the larynx (Fig 2–2). It can be directed inferiorly to one side until it can be seen entering the vocal fold and the injection can be made. Similarly the needle is directed to the opposite side and the injection can be made.

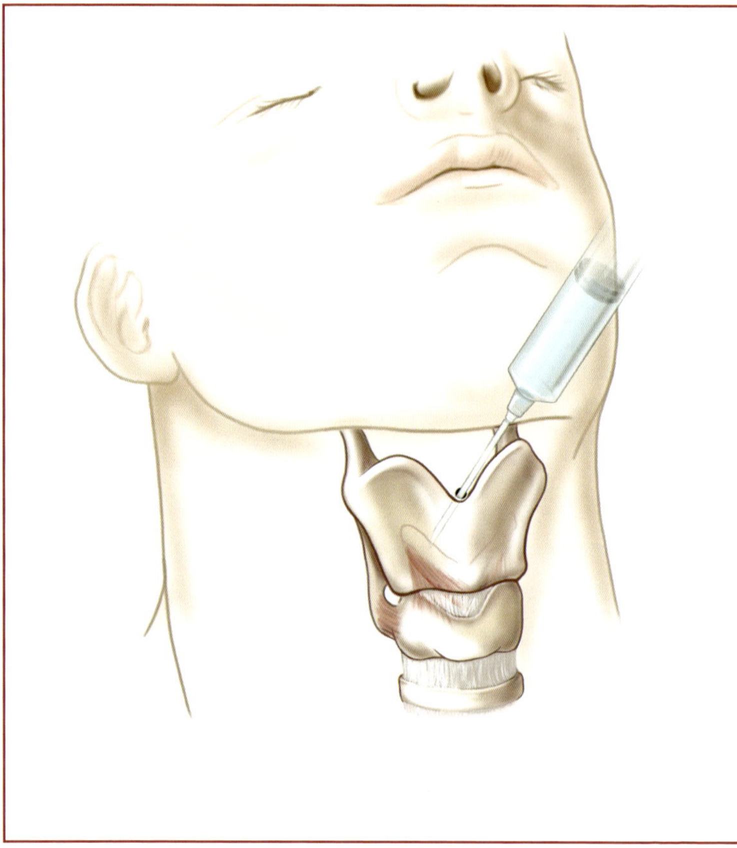

Figure 2–2

Injections From Above

There are two approaches to injecting Botox from above. The first is to have the patient hold their own tongue and a rigid endoscope can be passed through the mouth. A curved needle can then be passed into the vocal fold and injection made into the vocal folds (Fig 2–3). A similar approach can be made using a flexible scope. As these are longer needles, the volume of the needle needs to be taken into consideration.

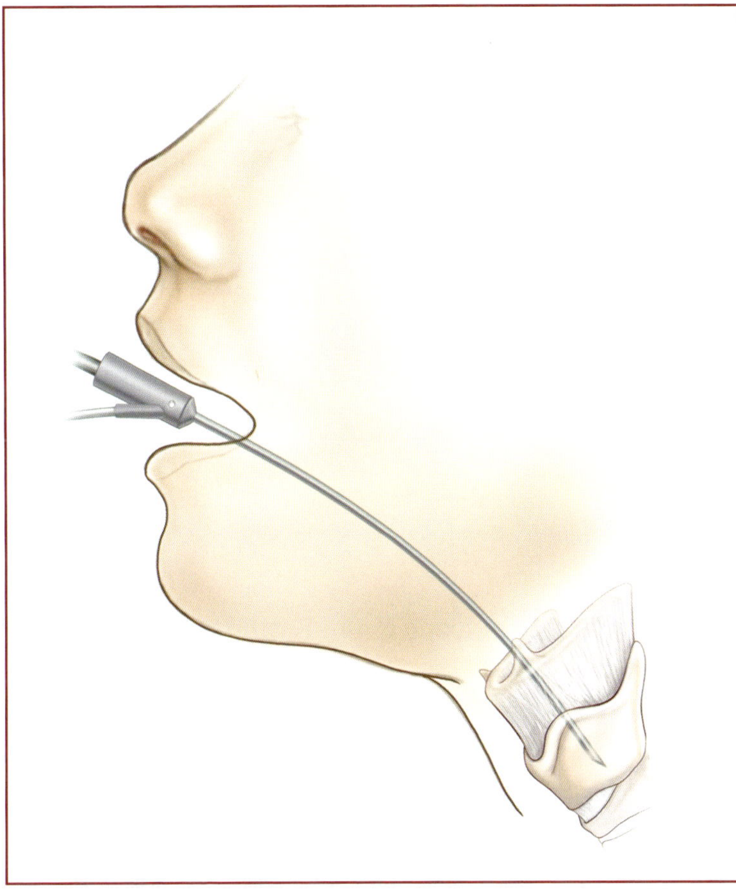

Figure 2–3

TECHNIQUES FOR ABDUCTOR SD

The success of Botox treatment in abductor SD is more variable than for adductor SD. The injections are made into the posterior cricoarytenoid muscle(s). Initially, a unilateral injection is typically performed. There have been concerns that bilateral injections at one sitting may result in poor abductor ability and may compromise the airway. With a unilateral injection 5 units is a good starting dose. Although most people note some improvement, a good response is seen in about 20% of patients.[1] They will usually require a second injection a month or so later and are often done in a staged fashion, with another 5 units injected at that time. It may be helpful to evaluate the larynx at the time of the second injection. As the injections are done blindly, there is a chance that the injection will be on the opposite side than expected and this should be detected on endoscopy, so that the subsequent injection can be performed on the more active side.

There have been increased interest in simultaneous bilateral posterior cricoarytenoid muscle injections and the safety has been well substantiated.[5] In these cases, the initial dose is approximately 2.5 units injected into each side.

Posterior-Lateral Approach to the Posterior Cricoarytenoid Muscle

The injections need to be performed with EMG guidance since the posterior cricoarytenoid muscle cannot be directly visualized. An injection is made in the skin at approximately the midpoint of the posterior aspect of the thyroid cartilage (Fig 2–4). The thyroid cartilage is rotated as much as is tolerated for patient comfort. The needle is passed through the skin until the posterior portion of the thyroid cartilage is encountered and the needle is then passed slightly inferiorly and medially until the cricoid cartilage is encountered and motor unit potentials are identified. The patient can then tighten their neck muscles to make sure that the needle is not in the strap muscle. They are then asked to sniff and EMG activity should increase verifying the position in the muscle. The injection is made. For a bilateral injection a similar approach could be made from the opposite side.

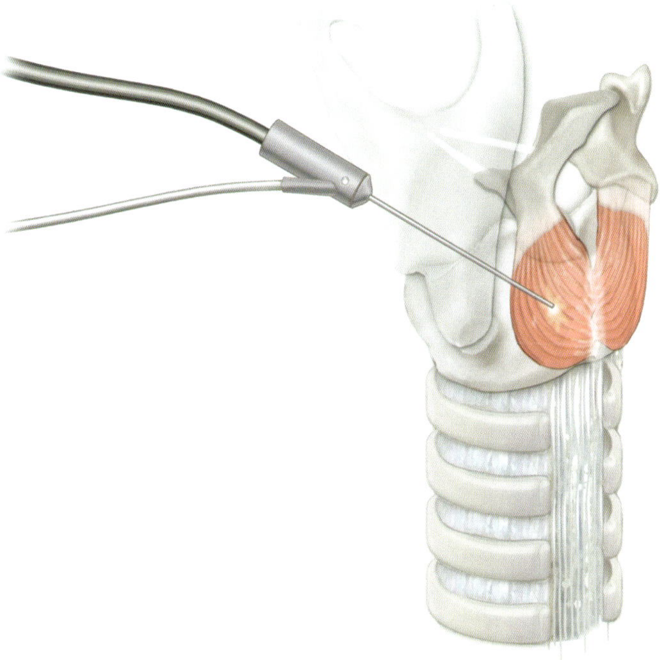

Figure 2–4

Injection Through the Cricoid Cartilage

This is a reasonable technique in patients who are relatively young and have little calcification of the thyroid cartilage. It is also more difficult in people with large larynges and thick cricoid cartilages. The needle is passed directly through both the anterior and posterior lamina of the cricoid cartilage, directed slightly laterally until the muscle is entered, and confirmed by EMG and the injection can be made (Fig 2–5). One of the problems

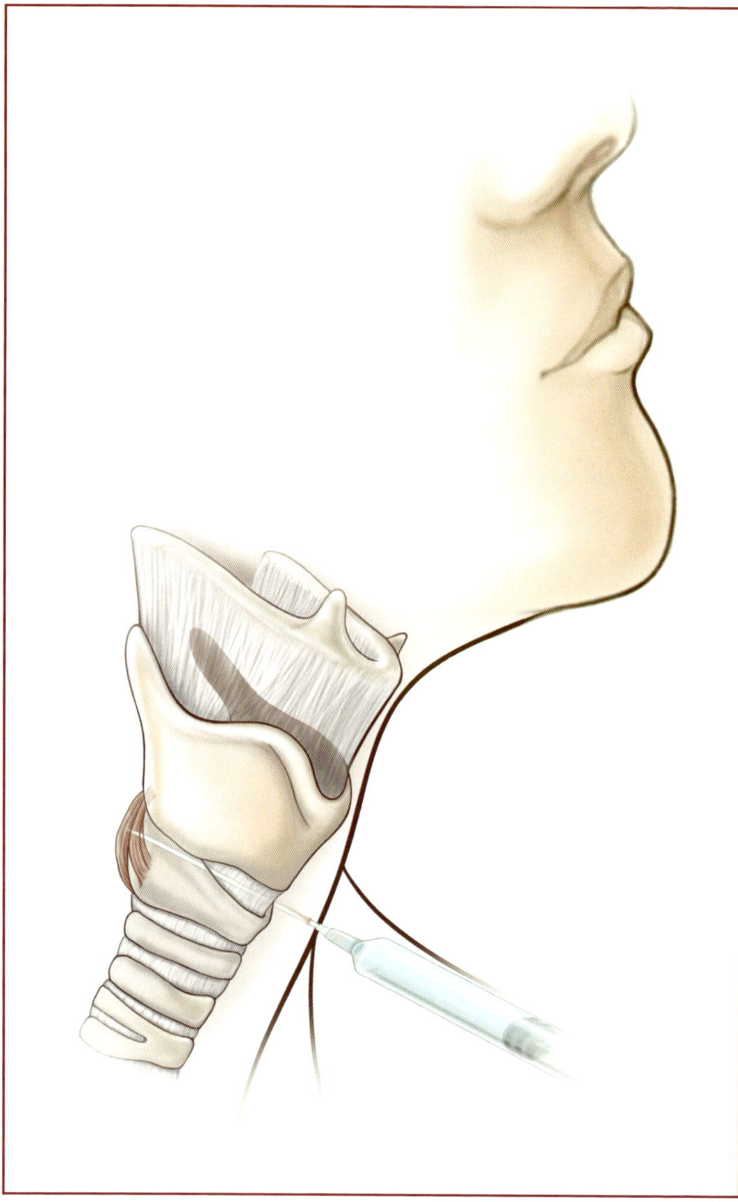

Figure 2–5

with this technique is that the needle can occasionally get plugged with cartilage, and it may be necessary to make a small push to eject some of the Botox or repeat the injection.

REFERENCES

1. Blitzer A, Brin MF, Stewart CF. Botulinum toxin management of spasmodic dysphonia (laryngeal dystonia): a 12-year experience in more than 900 patients. *Laryngoscope.* 1998;108:1435–1441.
2. Benninger MS, Gardner G, Grywalski C. The outcomes of botulinum toxin treatment for spasmodic dysphonia. *Arch Otolaryngol Head Neck Surg.* 2001;127:1083–1085.
3. Warfel JH. *The Head, Neck and Trunk: Muscles and Motor Points.* 4th ed. Philadelphia, PA: Lea and Febiger; 1978.
4. Woodson GE. Spasmodic dysphonia. In: Gates GE, ed. *Current Therapy in Otolaryngology Head and Neck Surgery.* St. Louis, MO: Mosby; 1998.
5. Klein A, Stong BC, Wise J, delGaudio JM, Hapner ER, Johns MM. Vocal outcome measures after bilateral posterior cricoarytenoid muscle botulinum toxin injections for abductor spasmodic dysphonia. *Otolaryngol Head Neck Surg.* 2008;139:421–423.

CHAPTER

3

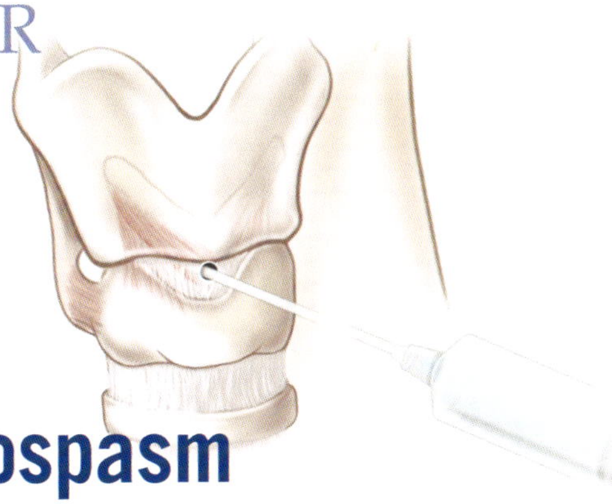

Blepharospasm

Michael S. Benninger

Essential blepharospasm is a focal involuntary cranial dystonia that is often progressive and bilateral.[1,2] Blepharospasm, like other dystonias, is characterized by forceful, uncontrollable and involuntary muscle contraction. In blepharospasm, the orbicularis oculi muscle is involved with tight and sometimes prolonged eyelid closure. It may be associated with other dystonias such as Meige syndrome or hemifacial spasm. As with other dystonias, medical and surgical therapy have proven largely unsuccessful. Beginning in 1976, botulinum toxin has been used to weaken extraocular muscles for the treatment of strabismus.[3]

Long-term successful treatment of essential blepharospasm and in blepharospasm association with hemifacial spasm and Meige syndrome was reported in the late 1980s. After injections with botulinum toxin, 97% of patient experienced sustained reduction of spasm for at least 2 weeks, beginning within 1 to 5 days after injection. Over 62% of patients felt that the injection was 75 to 100% effective.[1] Studies that looked at longer term follow-up of 5 years have shown satisfactory improvement of 85%, with an average effective time of 3½ months. There was no appreciable decrease in effectiveness after multiple injections.[4] Complications of botulinum therapy have been relatively minor and given the nature of the injections, they are temporary and localized. They have been reported to occur in as high as 23% of patients. Dry eye is the most common side effect and it occurs in 7.5% of cases. Ptosis occurs in 7.3% and photophobia in 2.5%, whereas diplopia happens in less than 1%.[1]

ANATOMIC CONSIDERATIONS

The orbicularis oculi is the primary sphincter of the eyelids. It can be divided into 3 portions: pretarsal, preseptal, and orbital. The muscles' vector of contraction is primarily horizontal, tightening the upper and lower lids and bringing their free edges together. The origin of the muscle is from the medial orbital margin, the palpebral part form the palpebral ligament, and the lacrimal part from the lacrimal bone. The orbital fibers arch over the upper lid and then return to the palpebral ligament, whereas the palpebral fibers converge at the lateral angle of the eye at the palpebral raphe. The lacrimal portion of the orbicularis oculi inserts into the medial portion of the lower and upper eyelids.[5]

TECHNIQUE

The technique of Botox injection into the extraocular muscles is performed with EMG guidance and under local anesthesia. Initial injection is generally 2.5 to 5.0 units intramuscularly in 2 separate areas in the medial and lateral portions of the preseptal orbicularis muscle of the upper eyelid and additional injections are made into the central and lateral aspect of the lower eyelid (Fig 3–1). As the orbicularis oculi muscle is relatively superficial a small needle (27-gauge needle) and a superficial injection, subcutaneously, are suggestions. If successful treatment is not effective at 5.0 units a site, then the dosage can be gradually increased.[1] Avoid injection to the midportion of the upper eyelid to avoid inadvertent diffusion into the levator palpebrae superiores as this may lead to unwanted ptosis. Other studies have used mean doses of 21 units but with a range of 5 to 50 units and 1 to 8 injection sites with a mean of 4.5 units. Averages of 5 units were given to each injection site.[6]

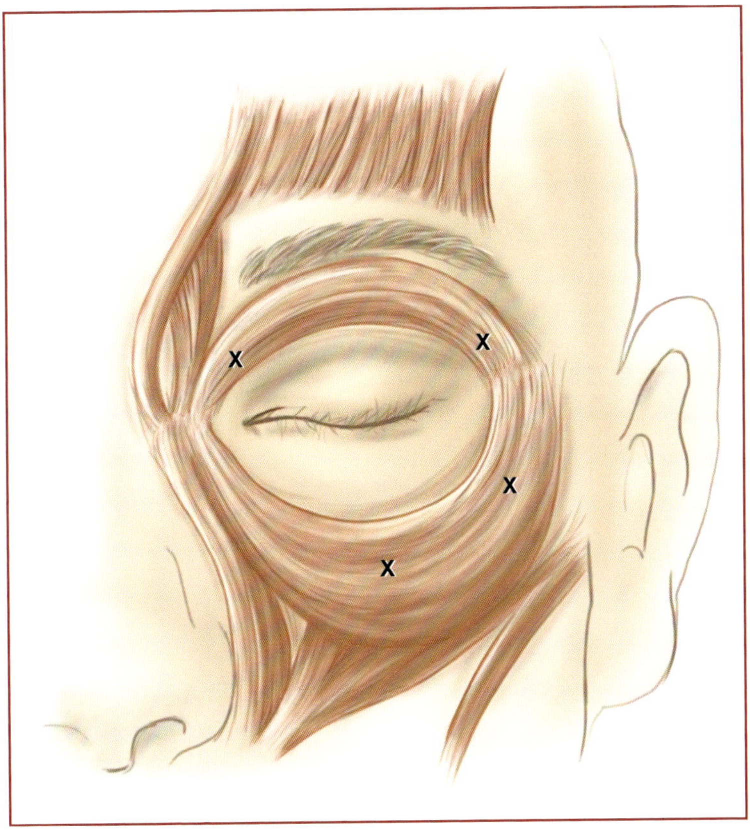

Figure 3–1

REFERENCES

1. Dutton JJ, Buckey EG. Long-term results and complications of botulinum A toxin in the treatment of blepharospasm. *Ophthalmology.* 1988;95:1529–1534.
2. Scott AB, Rosenbaum A, Collins CC. Pharmacologic weakening of extraocular muscles. *Invest Ophthalmol.* 1973;12:924–927.
3. Scott AB. Botulinum toxin injection into extracoular muscles as an alternative to strabismus surgery. *J Pediatr Ophthalmol Strabismus.* 1980;17:21–25.
4. Jankovic J, Brin MF. Therapeutic uses of boltulinum toxin. *N Engl J Med.* 1991;324:1186–1194.
5. Warfel JH. *The Head, Neck and Trunk: Muscles and Motor Points.* 4th ed. Philadelphia, PA: Lea and Febiger; 1978.
6. Scott AB, Kennedy RA, Stubbs HA. Botulinum A toxin injection as a treatment for blepharospasm. *Arch Ophthalmol.* 1985;103:347–350.

CHAPTER

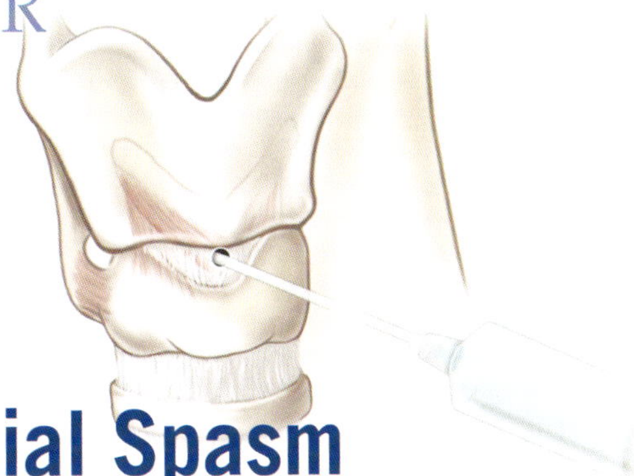

4

Hemifacial Spasm

Michael S. Benninger

Hemifacial spasm (HFS) is a focal facial disorder with segmental myoclonus of muscles innervated by the facial nerve. The disorder is predominantly unilateral although bilateral cases do occur. The hyperactivity can occur in any or all of the muscles innervated by the facial nerve including the orbicularis oculi, frontalis, zygomaticus, corrugator, and orbicularis. The initial presentation is often clonic contractions but will usually progress to more sustained tonic contractions of the muscles. Unlike the more classic dystonias described elsewhere in this book, there are multiple causes for the facial nerve hyperexcitability, involving either the facial nerve nucleus or the distal nerve. Overall, the etiology falls into 3 large categories: idiopathic HFS, compression lesions such as a tumor, vascular mass or bone disease, and noncompressive lesions such as multiple sclerosis, stroke, or meningitis. A large study performed by Wang and Jankovic evaluated 158 patients with HFS. The mean age at evaluation was 60 years with the mean age on onset of 48.5 years. Sixty-one percent of patients were women.[1] Underlying neurological disease is more common in the younger patient population, particularly those younger than 40 years of age. A workup, usually including an MRI, should be performed to look for primary causes.

With early idiopathic HFS and mild noncompressive lesions, medications such as carbamazepine, baclofen, or benzodiazepines may be effective. In most cases, however, the effect of the medication may not be adequate or the side effects may be significant. In most cases, therefore, botulinum toxin injections become an excellent alternative and some feel may be the treatment of choice.[2–4]

ANATOMIC CONSIDERATIONS

Hemifacial spasm involves the muscles of facial expression, largely innervated by the facial nerve. Although there are 5 major branches of the facial nerve (temporalis, zygomatic, buccal, mandibular, and cervical), from an anatomic standpoint there are also smaller branches that should be considered related to the functional distribution to the muscles of facial movement (posterior auricular, digastric, and stylohyoid). There are multiple muscles that are either completely or partially innervated by the facial nerve and a review of the anatomy of each of these is beyond the goals of this book, but they are mentioned so that they can be considered when evaluating patients with HMS: occipital-frontalis, auriculares, temporoparietal, orbicularis oculi, currugator, procerus, compressor nares, dilator nares, depresor septi, levator labii superioris, risorius, depressor labii inferioris, depressor anguli oris, mentalis, orbiculoris oris, buccinator, platysma, digastric, stylohyoid, and stapedius. Table 4–1 describes the distribution of muscle involvement by symptoms and by clinical examination in patients with HFS as identified by Wang and Jankovik.[1]

When considering botulinum injections for HMS, usually the larger muscle groups are the more significant in the degree

Table 4–1. *Symptom Location and Anatomic Distribution in HFS*[1]

Location	Site of Onset by History (%)	Affected Site by Exam (%)
Frontalis	0 (0)	38 (24)
Orbicularis oculi	142 (90)	152 (94)
Eyebrow	4 (3)	8 (5)
Zygomatic	0 (0)	87 (55)
Cheek	18 (11)	8 (5)
Paranasal	2 (1)	34 (22)
Perioral	15 (9)	99 (63)
Chin/mentalis	0 (0)	33 (21)
Platysma	0 (0)	48 (33)
Other	2 (1)	5 (2)

of symptoms. In addition the orbicularis oculi is almost always involved, and is often the first muscle where the spasms are noticeable. This can lead initially to a diagnosis of blepahrospasm, until the other muscle become more noticeable.

INJECTION TECHNIQUE

As the orbicularis oculi is the most commonly involved muscle, usually it will need to be injected. We take the same approach that we take for essential blepharospasm. The technique of Botox injection into the extraocular muscles is performed with EMG guidance and under local anesthesia. Initial injection is generally 2.5 to 5.0 units intramuscularly in 2 separate areas in the medial and lateral portions of the preseptal orbicularis muscle of the upper eyelid and additional injections are made into the central and lateral aspect of the lower eyelid (Fig 4–1). As the orbicularis oculi muscle is relatively superficial a small needle (27-gauge needle) and a superficial injection, subcutaneously, are suggestions. If successful treatment is not effective at 5.0 units a site, then the dosage can be gradually increased.[5] Avoid injection to the midportion of the upper eyelid to avoid

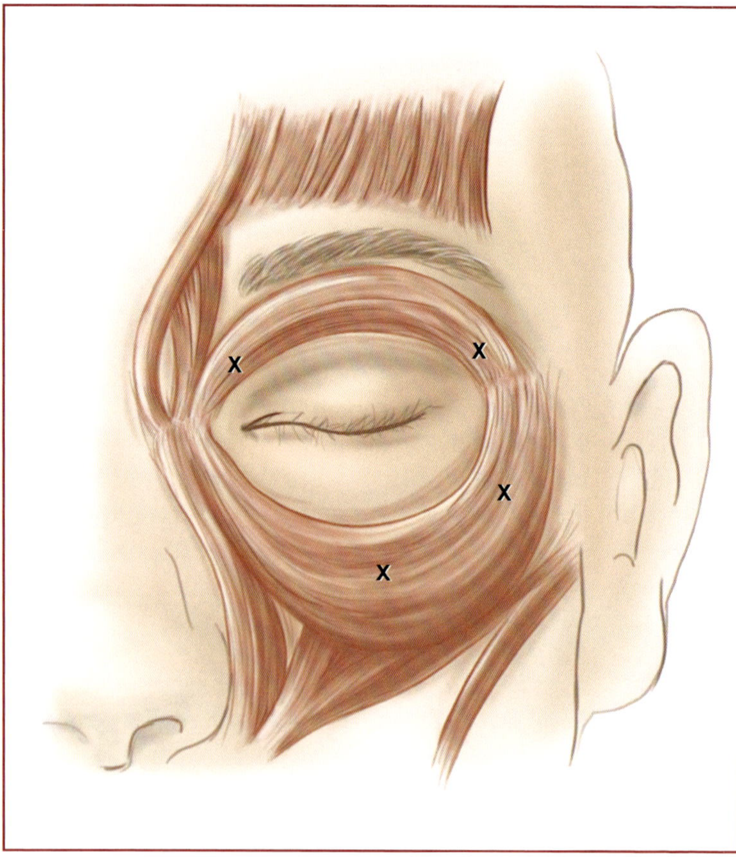

Figure 4–1

inadvertent diffusion into the levator palpebrae superiores as this may lead to unwanted ptosis.

As the involvement of the other muscle groups is not consistent, the determination of where to inject will depend on the most active muscles involved on clinical evaluation (see Table 4–1). Commonly involved muscles are the frontalis, the muscles along the zygoma, the perioral muscles, and the platysma. EMG is typically used unless there is gross muscle contraction where position of the needle can be confirmed. For the frontalis, 2 to 3 injections on the one side can be made in different locations with a dose of 4 to 5 units of Botox per site (Fig 4–2). For the perioral injections both the lip elevators (zygomaticus major and minor), the oral sphincter (orbicularis oris), and the lateral lip depressors (the depressor labii inferioris and the depressor anguli oris) may need to be injected (Fig 4–3). Three to five units of Botox can be injected into these sites. The platysma can be more difficult and small doses of Botox (2–3 units) may need to be distributed over a few sites of the active muscle (Fig 4–4).

A large study was performed by Wang and Jankovic[1] in 84 patients where Botox was used to treat their HFS and where they had long enough follow-up to assess outcomes. The mean number of visits where the patients came for injections was 5.5 with a range of 1 to 28 visits. Patients were followed for 3 to 13 years The average amount of Botox injected was 33 units, with a range from 5 to 100. Clinical benefit began anywhere from 0 to 45 days after injection with an average of 5.4 days after. The total duration of benefit averaged 18 weeks. Eighty percent of the patients had a peak effect of 4 (marked improvement in severity and function), and 15% had a score of 3 (moderate improvement in severity and function). Only 2 patients (1%) reported no improvement with the first injection and did not return for a follow-up treatment. Although 70% of patients reported at least one side effect of the injections, they were felt to be mild and none were considered disabling. Facial weakness (30%), lid weakness (26%), and ptosis (20%) were the most common side effects, whereas dry eye and diplopia were less common.[1]

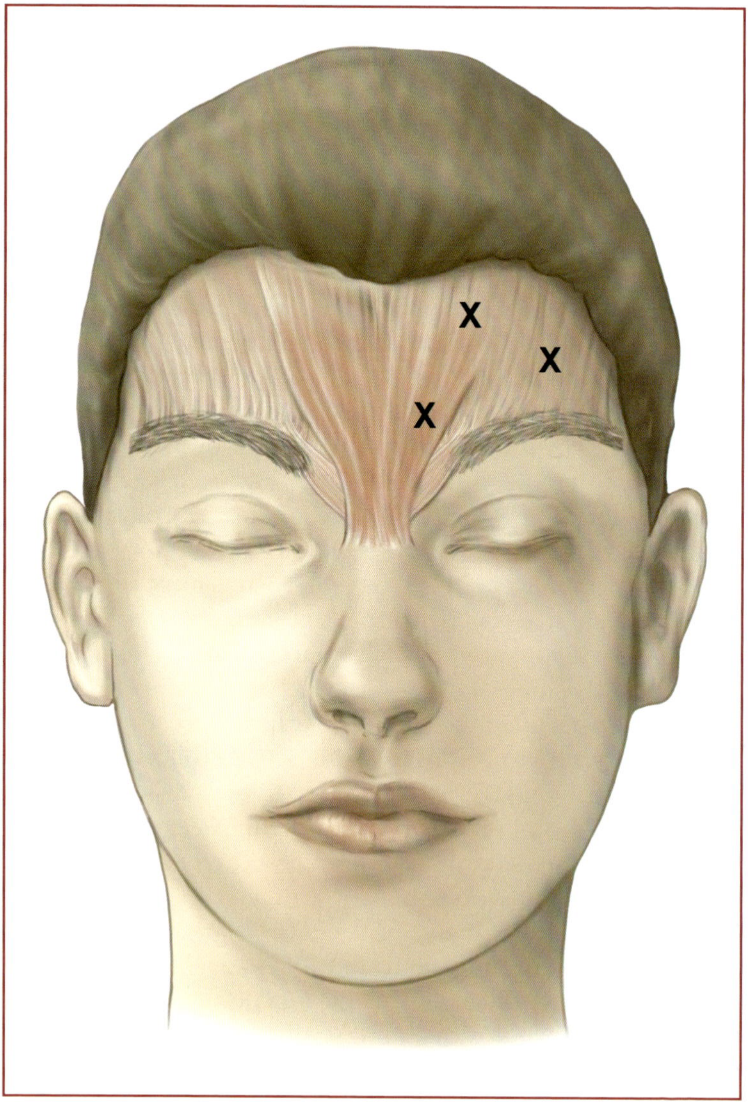

Figure 4–2

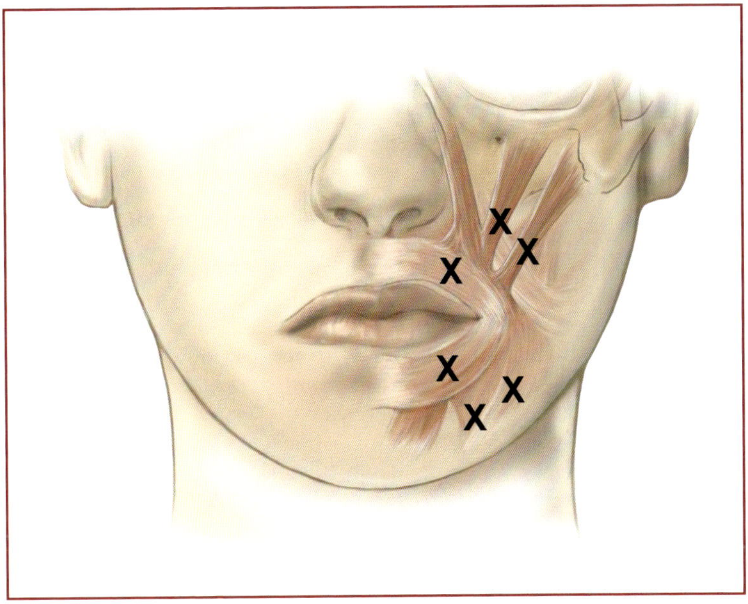

Figure 4–3

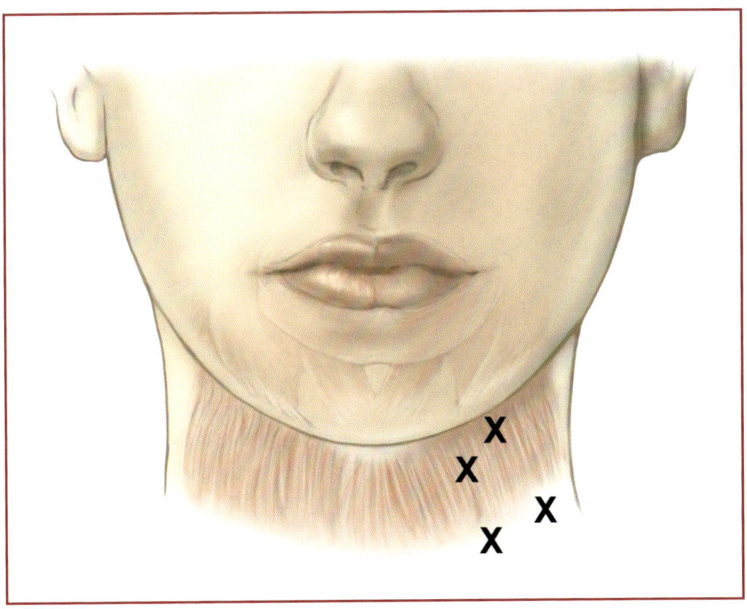

Figure 4–4

REFERENCES

1. Wang A, Jankovic J. Hemifacial spasm: clinical findings and treatment. *Muscle Nerve.* 1998;21:1740–1747.
2. Jankovic J, Brin MF. Therapeutic uses of boltulinum toxin. *N Engl J Med.* 1991;324:1186–1194.
3. Jankovic J, Schwartz K, Donovan DT. Botulinum toxin treatment of cranial-cervical dystonia, spasmodic dysphonia, other focal dystonias and hemifacial spasm. *J Neurol Neurosurg Psychiatry.* 1990;53:633–639.
4. Mauriello JA, Leone T, Dhillon S, et al. Treatment choices of 119 patients with hemifacial spasm over 11 years. *Clin Neurol Neurosurg.* 1996;98:213–216.
5. Dutton JJ, Buckey EG. Long-term results and complications of botulinum A toxin in the treatment of blepharospasm. *Ophthalmology.* 1988;95:1529–1534.

CHAPTER

5

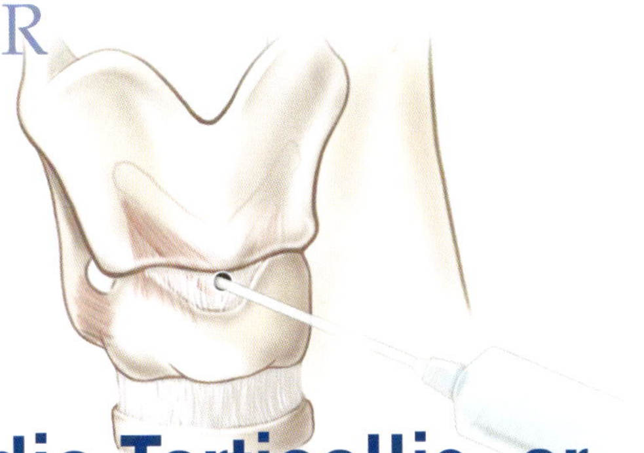

Spasmodic Torticollis, or Cervical Dystonia

Michael S. Benninger

Spasmodic torticollis, or cervical dystonia, is a focal dystomia of the muscles of the neck and shoulder. The symptoms are painful contraction of the neck musculature, often with turning of the neck in the direction of the most significantly contracting muscles, often the sternocleidomastoid muscle. Laterocollis (tilting) seems to be the most common isolated type and it is associated with the head bending laterally, moving the ear toward the ipsilateral shoulder. Retrocollis is associated with extension of the neck and upward extension of the chin. Anterocollis results in a forward flexion, deviating the chin downward toward the chest. These can occur in isolation or in any combination of these deviations. Similar to other focal dystonias, the cause is unknown, medical treatment is largely ineffective, and long-term effectiveness of any therapy has not been shown. Although surgery is an option, the effects of transaction of these large muscles, in themselves, may be disabling. Botulinum toxin has been shown to be an effective treatment for many patients with torticollis.[1–3]

ANATOMIC CONSIDERATIONS

The sternocleidomastoid muscle is the predominant muscle that is injected for torticollis. The origin has a sternal head that attaches to anterior surface of the manubrium and a clavicular head that attaches to the medial upper third of the clavicle. The insertion is at the lateral surface of the mastoid process and the lateral half of the superior nuchal line of the occiput.[4] The splenius capitus muscle is a posterior neck muscle with an origin from the lower half of the ligamentum nuchae and the spine of the 7th cervical and upper thoracic vertebrae. It inserts into the mastoid process and the lateral half of the superior nuchal line of the occiput and the transverse process of the upper cervical vertebrae. The trapezius muscle is a large fan-shaped posterior neck muscle that originates at the occipital bone medial-superiorly, from the ligamentum nuchae, the spinous process of the seventh cervical, and all the thoracic vertebrae. It fans out and superiorly inserts into the posterior border of the calicle and more inferiorly in the spine of the scapula and the medial acromion.[4]

TECHNIQUE

The muscles that are generally injected are the sternocleidomastoid (Fig 5–1), trapezius (Fig 5–2), and splenius capitus (Fig 5–3) and the muscles that are thought to be most active are chosen for injection. A careful evaluation of the muscles in various head positions will help to identify the most involved muscles. EMG guidance is recommended, aspirating the needle prior to injection in order to ensure that it is not in a vessel. With large muscles like the sternocleidomastoid muscle where the position of the needle can be ascertained by physical examination, EMG may not be necessary, although it is usually helpful.

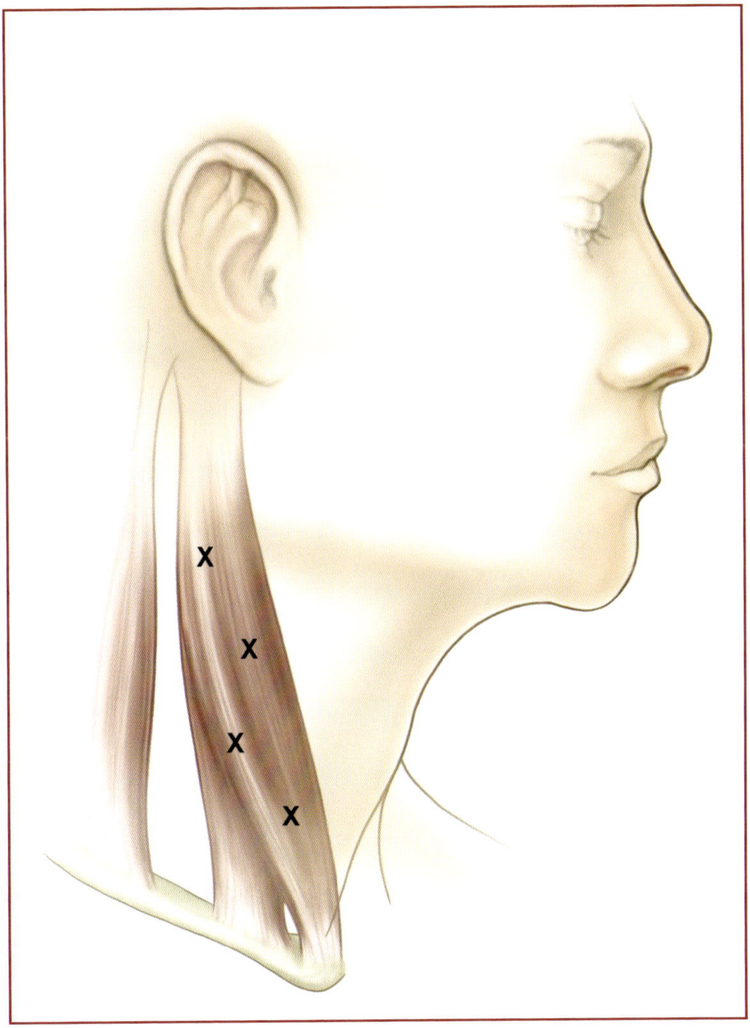

Figure 5–1

Usually between 2 and 4 of these muscles are injected, although more injections may be performed into 2 to 8 sites per muscle with larger numbers of injection sites into larger

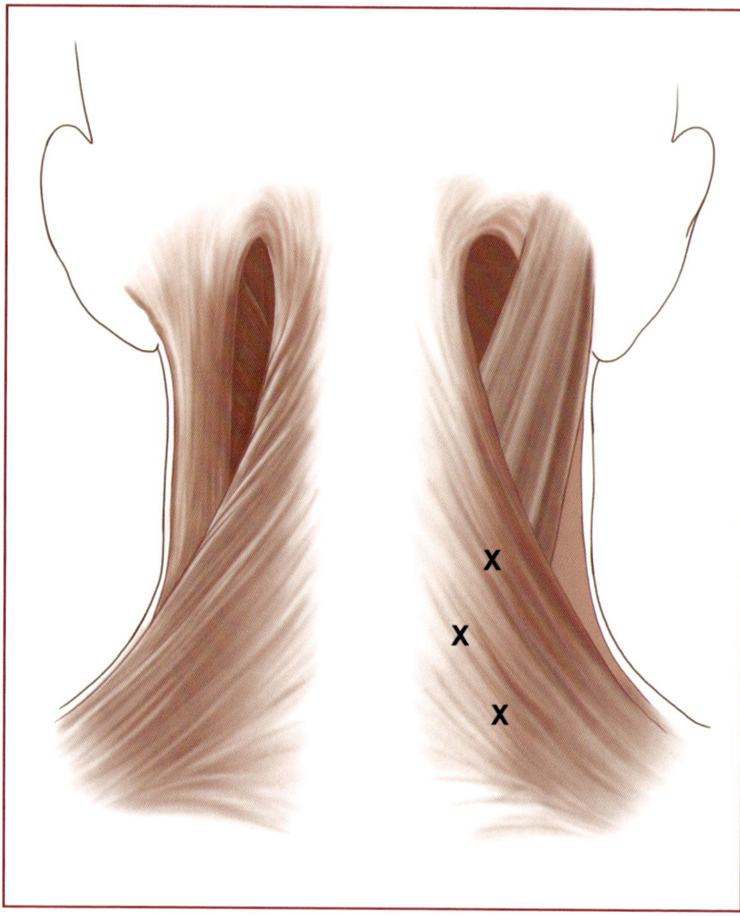

Figure 5–2

muscles or into broad areas of increased muscle activity (see Figs 5–1, 5–2, and 5–3). Randomized trials have shown that effectiveness can be achieved with an intermediate dose of 100 to 140 units of Botox spread among the muscles injected, and between 20 to 90 units per muscle.[2,3] Doses as high as 280 units have been reported.[2] There is potential for significant variabil-

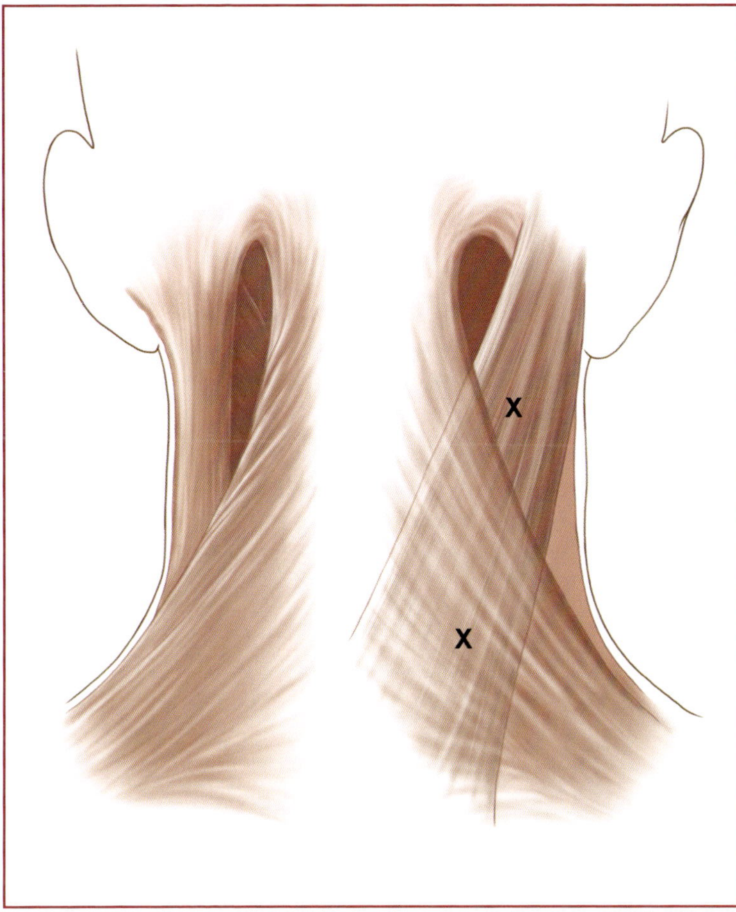

Figure 5–3

ity in the dosing and which muscles are chosen for injections, and therefore there is the potential for variability in the results. In addition, it may take a few injections with a single patient before the best muscles and optimal results are recognized. The correct dose for each muscle and each patient therefore must be individualized. A reasonable approach is to use a median dose of around 120 units and increase up to 250 units if unsuccessful with the lower doses.[2] Despite this variability, ultimate success rates of around 75% are expected.[1–3]

REFERENCES

1. Tsui JKC, Eisen A, Stoessl AJ, Calne S, Calne DB. Double-blind study of botulinum toxin in spasmodic torticollis. *Lancet*. 1986;2:245–247.
2. Gelb DJ, Lowenstein DH, Aminoff MJ. Controlled trial of botulinum toxin injections in the treatment of spasmodic torticollis. *Neurology*. 1989;39:80–84.
3. Greene P, kang U, Fahn S, Brin M, Moskowitz C, Flaster E. Double-blind, placebo-controlled trial of botulinum toxin injections for the treatment of spasmodic torticollis. *Neurology*. 1990;40:1213–1218.
4. Warfel JH. *The Head, Neck and Trunk: Muscles and Motor Points*. 4th ed. Philadelphia, PA: Lea and Febiger; 1978.

CHAPTER

6

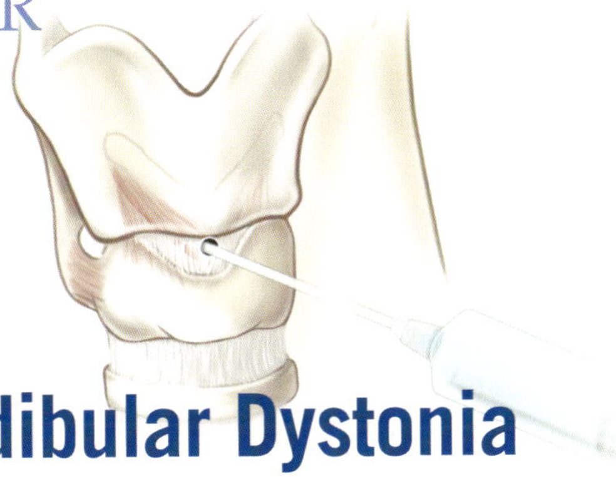

Oromandibular Dystonia

Michael S. Benninger

Oromandibular dystonia (OMD) results in involuntary repetitive spasms of the muscles of mastication, tongue, and sometimes the pharynx resulting in uncontrolled jaw and tongue movements. It is one of the many cranial-cervical dystonias that may involve the musculature of the mastication, face, tongue, pharynx, larynx, neck, and periorbita. OMD is often classified related to the visible functional result such as jaw opening, jaw closing, jaw deviation, and/or tongue protrusion type.[1] Meige syndrome is a variant of OMD which is when these OMD symptoms are also found in conjunction with blephorospasm. OMD can lead to a number of uncomfortable symptoms such as bruxism, temporomandibular joint disorders, difficulty eating, chewing, or swallowing, and fragmented articulation and speech. The facial spasms that occur are not only uncomfortable they often lead to significant embarrassment for the patient.[2] Botulinum toxin has been used successfully in treating both focal and segmental dystonia.[1–3]

ANATOMIC CONSIDERATIONS

There are a number of muscles that are important in consideration of injection for OMD. The action of these muscles is listed in Table 6–1. The internal (medial) pterygoid has its origin in the pyramidal process of the palatine bone, the medial surface of the pterygoid plate, and tuberosity of the maxilla. It inserts in the medial surface of the ramus and angle of the mandible. The external (lateral) pterygoid muscle has its origins in the infratemproal surface of the greater wing of the sphenoid and the lateral surface of the lateral pterygoid plate. It inserts in the front of the neck of the mandibular condyle and capsule of the mandibular joint. The masseter muscle arises from the anterior two-thirds of the lower border and the medial surface of the zygomatic arch and inserts on the coronoid process of the mandible, and the upper half of the ramus and angle of

Table 6–1. *Muscles and Their Primary Actions*[1]

Muscle	Primary Action
Anterior digastric	Jaw opening, tongue elevation
External pterygoids	Jaw opening, jaw deviation, protrusion
Genioglossus	Jaw opening, tongue protrusion
Geniohyoid	Jaw opening
Hyoglossus	Jaw opening, tongue protrusion
Mylohyoid	Jaw opening, tongue elevation
Masseter	Jaw closing
Temporalis	Jaw closing
Internal pterygoid	Jaw closing

the mandible. The temporalis muscle is a broad, paired, fan-shaped muscle on the lateral sides of the head. The function of the temporalis muscle is to elevate the jaw, clench the teeth and retract the mandible. The muscle originates at the floor of the temporal fossa and in the temporalis fascia. It inserts in the anterior boarder of the ramus and the anterior boarder of the coronoid process of the mandible. The posterior belly of the digastric has its origin at the mastoid notch of the temporal bone whereas the anterior belly begins at the digastric fossa of the mandible. Both bellies insert by and intermediate tendon which passes through the stylohyoid muscle.[4]

TECHNIQUE

The key to treating OMD with botulinum toxin is a careful evaluation of the muscles that are the most involved. In addition as described by Cultrara et al, "it is imperative to have an in-depth knowledge of the origin, insertion, and action of the muscles potentially involved in OMD. Delivering precise injections will help maximize therapeutic benefit while minimizing morbidity. In our practice, we routinely use electromyography (EMG) guidance to confirm needle placement and muscle activity before injection."[1] The focus of the injection is mostly directed at the muscles of mastication including the internal and external pterygoid, the temporalis, the masseter and the digastric muscles. Cultrara et al have presented an excellent short summary of the action of each of the key muscles involved in OMD and this is presented in Table 6–1.[1]

The treatment is usually performed with EMG guidance although it is possible to identify the muscles by anatomic guidelines, particularly for the masseter, external pterygoid, and temporalis muscles. EMG allows for quicker and more reliable identification of the muscles and activation of the jaw opening or closing behavior with increased EMG activity will help to ensure that the appropriate muscles are injected. OMD is a challenging disorder to treat and there is often some trial and error before the best muscles are chemically denervated with botulinum toxin. Some advocate for a trial with a local anesthetic prior to injection but we have found that the primary muscles to be injected can be determined by paying attention to the patient's description of which muscles they seem to feel are the most significant, and careful physical examination and observation.

Botulinum toxin injection is not standardized but instead is determined on a case by case basis, depending on the number of muscles involved and the degree of hyperactivity. Although we vary our initial injection of Botox based on the severity of the spasm and the number of muscles involved, good starting points have been reported.[1] Under most circumstances we start with these doses: temporalis muscle 25 units, masseter 20 units, external pterygoid 15 units, anterior digastric 10 units, and internal pterygoid 10 units. Some people use 20 units in each muscle. In most cases, only a few muscles need to be injected, although greater caution should be exercised when injecting greater numbers of muscles. Bilateral injection of multiple muscles should also be performed with care. For example, with jaw closing dystonia, injections of bilateral masseter, internal pterygoids, and temporalis muscles may leave the patient without the ability to close the mouth or chew. Overaggressive injection in the submental region for jaw opening dystonia may result in diffusion into the intrinsic muscles of the tongue with potential dysphagia or dysarthria.

The masseter and temporalis muscles are initially injected for jaw closing dystonias. The pterygoids are more difficult to reach, are more uncomfortable to inject and harder to ensure appropriate location of the injection. Local anesthetic is generally not used as the multiple injection sites are needed and local anesthesia injection in multiple sites is as uncomfortable as the injections themselves. The temporalis is relatively easy to identify. A 27-gauge needle is passed through the skin in the area of the bulk of the muscle as it fans out over the temporal region of the skull. If EMG is used, the patient is asked to clench their teeth and brisk increase in muscle activity ensures proper placement. The 25 units are equally distributed over 3 to 4 injection sites (Fig 6–1). If EMG is not used, the needle is

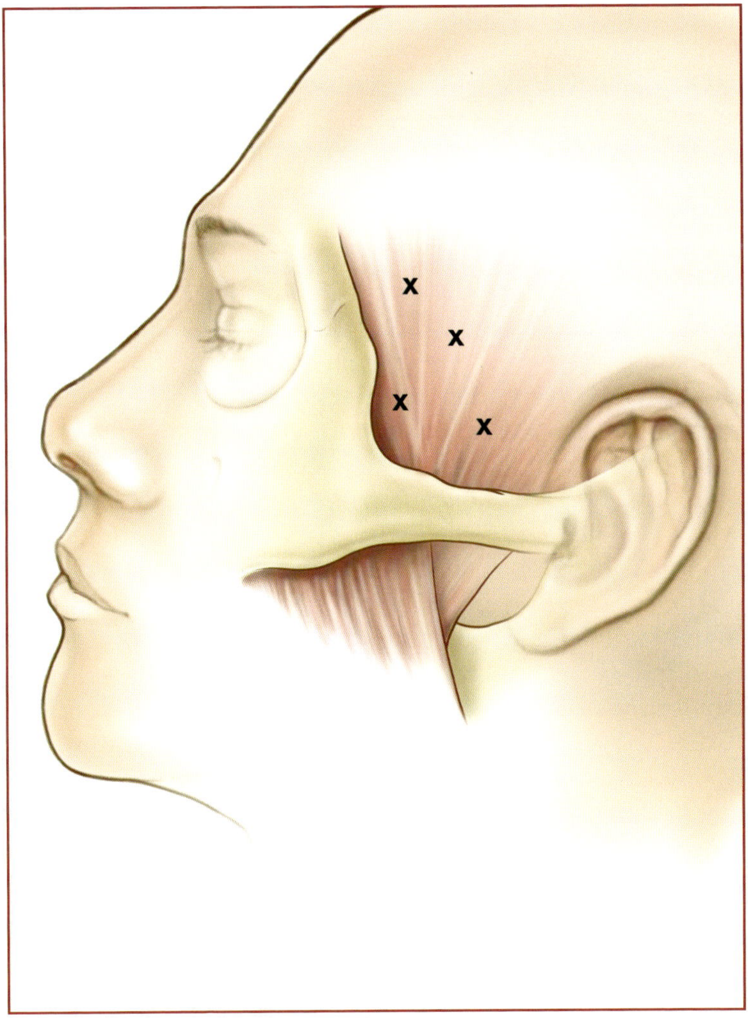

Figure 6–1

passed until the skull is encountered and then withdrawn a mm or 2 and the injection is made. In most patients with OMD, we tend to repeat the procedure on the other side, unless there is clear evidence of unilaterality. The masseter is reached by passing the needle through the skin over the angle of the mandible and then passed until the bone is encountered, where it can be withdrawn slightly. The location is confirmed with increased EMG activity with teeth clenching. We prefer to aspirate the needle in this location to prevent the minimal likelihood of intravascular injection. The 20 units are distributed equally in 3 to 4 sites in the muscle (Fig 6–2). Although this can also be performed without EMG, the overlying parotid gland and the thicker tissue of the lateral face make this more difficult. The other masseter is usually also injected.

The combined injections of the masseters and the temporalis muscles is usually sufficient to provide good relief of symptoms while internal pterygoid activity will allow for some jaw closing. On rare occasions we find that one or both internal pterygoids also need to be injected. We prefer to try one first and proceed with the other if there is not adequate improvement. The injection of the internal pterygoids needs to be done with EMG guidance. The needle is passed along the inner surface of the mandible beginning in the middle of the mandible just anterior to the angle of the jaw. Local anesthesia to the skin in this location may be helpful, as on occasion the needle may need to be placed more than once and it can reduce the discomfort of passing the needle through the skin. The needle is directed superiorly along the ramus of the mandible while asking the patient to clench their teeth, until brisk activity is encountered. We then ask them to relax and reclench to ensure placement. In this location, we also aspirate to confirm proper placement and ensure that the needle does not move into a vessel. Once the location is confirmed, a single injection of 10 units is delivered (Fig 6–3).

In our experience the success of injections for jaw opening dystonias is not as predictable as that for jaw closing dystonia treatment. For jaw opening dystonias, the anterior belly of

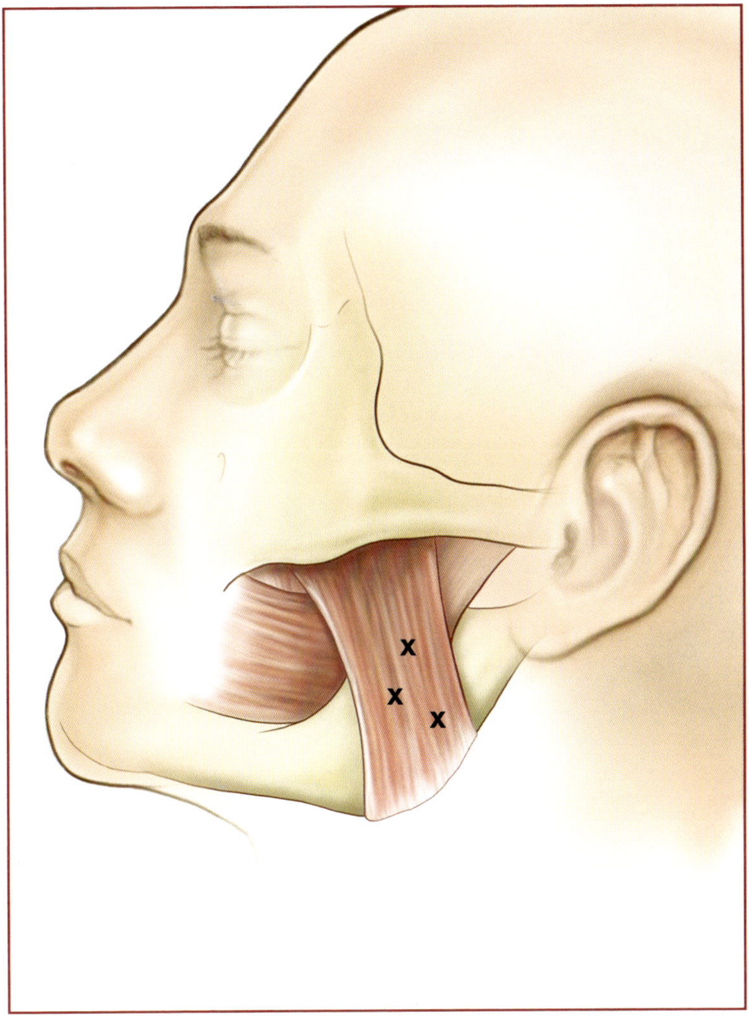

Figure 6–2

the digastric and the internal pterygoid muscles are injected. Although other muscles, such as the mylohyoid, hyoglossus, and even the primary muscles of the tongue, may be involved in either jaw opening dystonia or in those patients with tongue

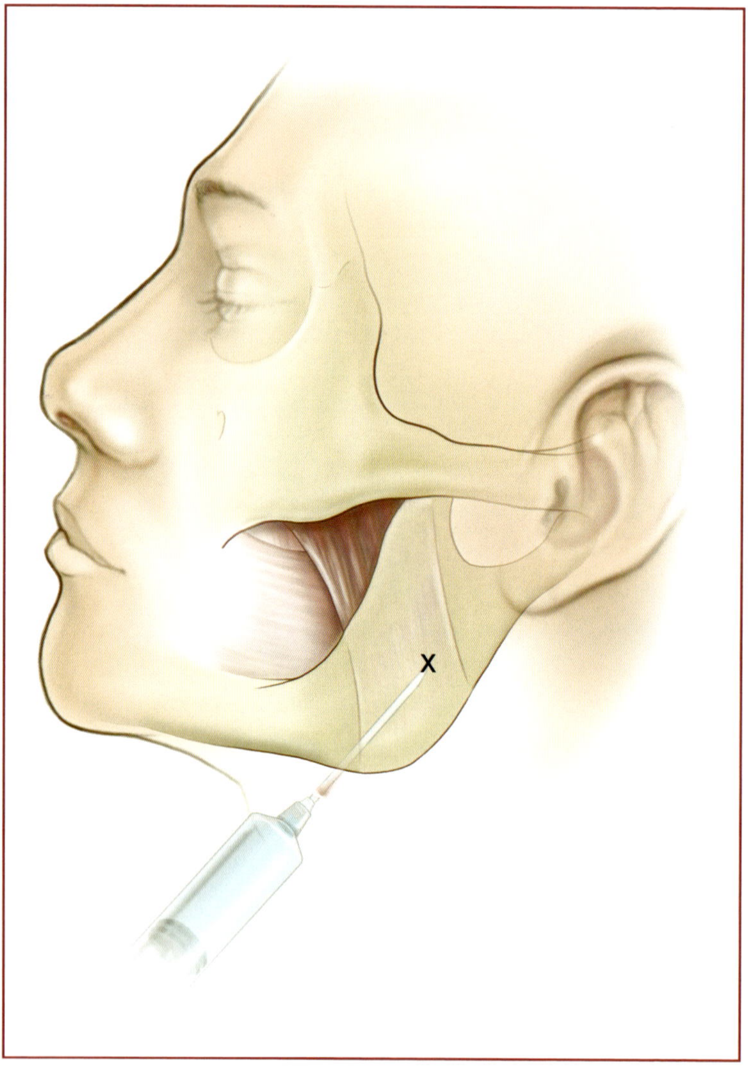

Figure 6–3

thrusting, the risks of significant functional problems with tongue motion, dysarthria, and dysphagia with injection of these muscles has led us to focusing on the digastric and internal pterygoid muscles. Particular care should be taken to ensure that the Botox is reconstituted with a low volume of fluid for the anterior belly of the digastric injection to prevent diffusion of the botulinum toxin into the adjacent muscles.

Similar to the external pterygoid, the internal pterygoid is injected with EMG guidance. The internal pterygoid is reached by having the patient open their mouth, and the needle is passed through the mucosa of the lingual buccal sulcus near the retromolar trigone of the maxilla. The needle is passed posteriorly past the peterygoid plate and in the direction of the condyle of the mandible. The patient is asked to open and close the mouth slightly and from side to side until an obvious increase in EMG activity is encountered. A single dose of 15 units is delivered. A similar injection is then made on the other side (Fig 6–4).

The anterior belly of the digastric is reached by passing the needle through the skin in the submental area a few millimeters laterally to the midline and approximately halfway between the mandible and the hyoid bone. To prevent diffusion into the tongue musculature it is recommended that EMG be used for guidance. The patient is then asked to open their mouth widely until brisk EMG activity is encountered. 10 units of botulinum toxin is then injected either in one or two locations along the muscle. In a similar fashion the other side is injected by passing the needle a few mm lateral to the midline on the other side (Fig 6–5).

As mentioned earlier, the success of botulinum toxin injections for OMD are often unpredictable and it may take 2 to 3 sessions to obtain the best results. Patients should be cautioned that this may be the case at the time of the first injection. They should also be informed of the potential side effects related to injections of too high a dose of toxin or into the wrong muscles. These include but are not limited to dysphagia, dysarthria, difficulty chewing, drooling, or opening or closing the mouth.

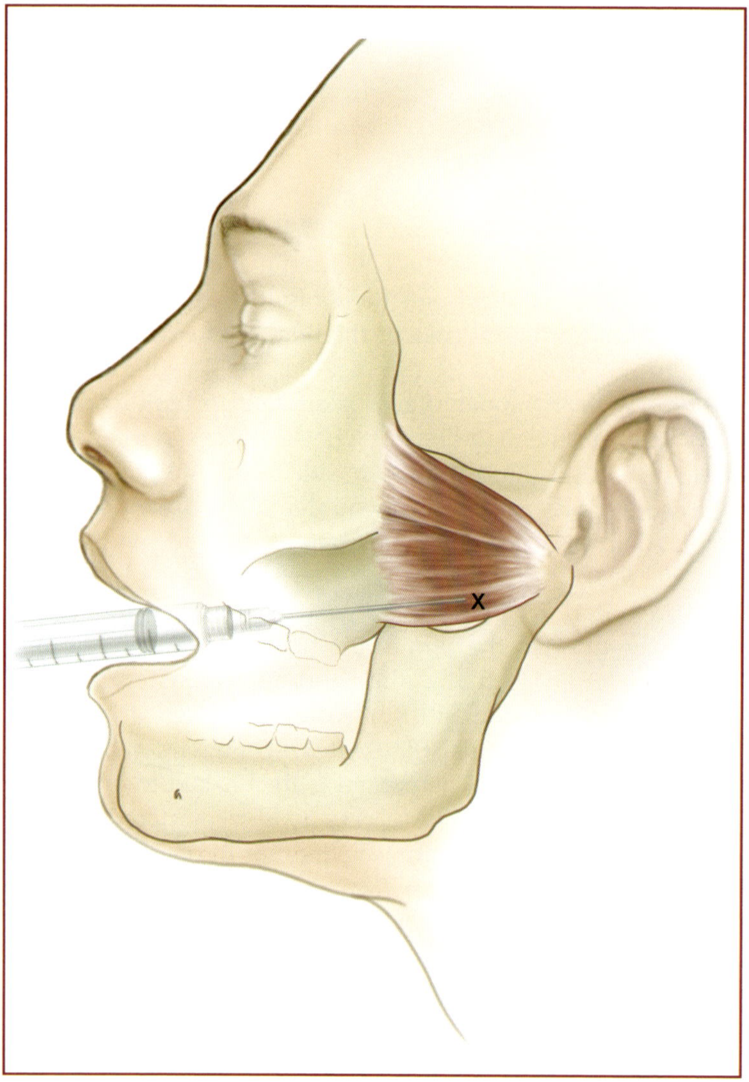

Figure 6–4

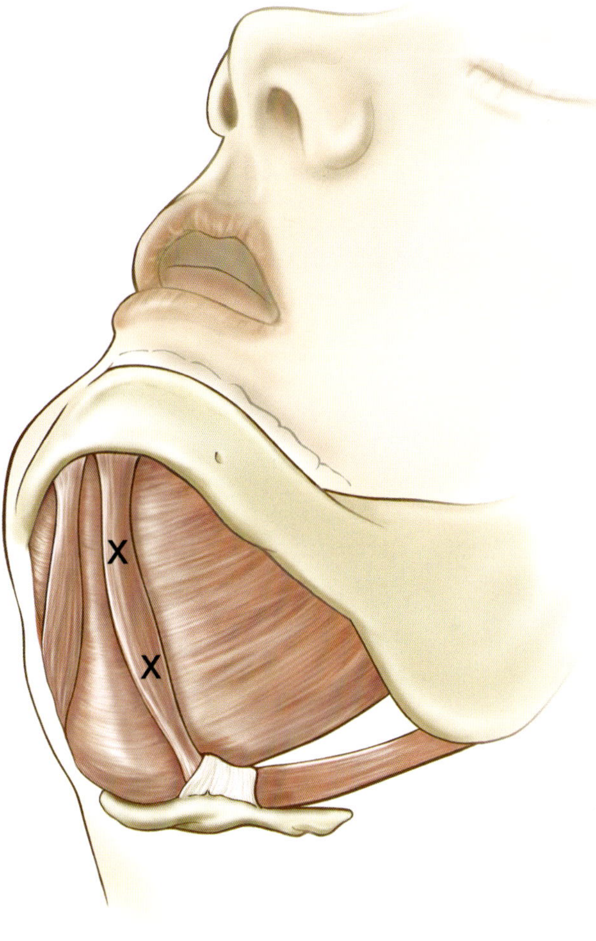

Figure 6–5

REFERENCES

1. Cultrara A, Chitkara A, Blitzer A. Botulinum toxin injections for the treatment of oromandibular dystonia. *Oper Tech Otolaryngol Head Neck Surg*. 2004;15:97–102.
2. Bhattacharyya N, Tarsy D. Impact on quality of life of botulinum toxin treatments for spasmodic dysphonia and oromandibular dystonia. *Arch Otolaryngol Head Neck Surg*. 2001;127:389–392.
3. Tan EK, Jankovic J. Botulinum toxin A in patients with oromandibular dystonia: long-term follow-up. *Neurology*. 1999;53:2102–2107.
4. Warfel JH. *The Head, Neck and Trunk: Muscles and Motor Points*. 4th ed. Philadelphia, PA: Lea and Febiger; 1978.

SECTION

II

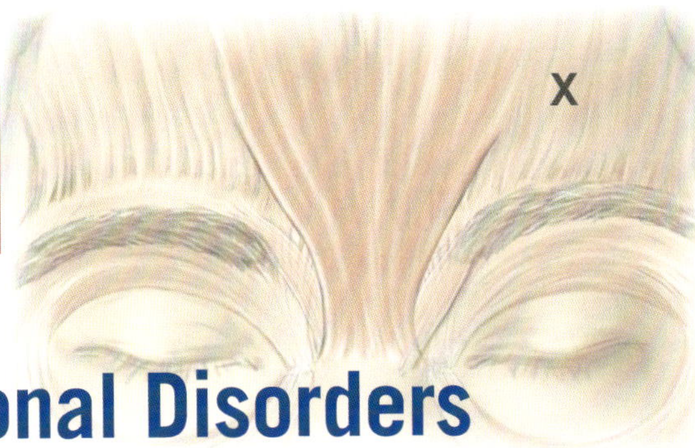

Functional Disorders

Michael S. Benninger

The following chapters are grouped together under the heading of functional disorders. Although there are multiple areas and etiologies, we have classified them as functional in that they do not have a common cause or diagnosis and they impact normal function. There are multiple functional disorders of the head and neck that may benefit from botulinum toxin treatment. Unlike the previous section of dystonias, functional disorders often are the sequellae of treatment of other head and neck disorders and may particularly follow surgical treatment. Although they are disparate in both causes and symptoms, it is reasonable to consider them together as their treatment is designed to improve function and localized symptoms such as dysphagia or sialorrhea.

CHAPTER

7

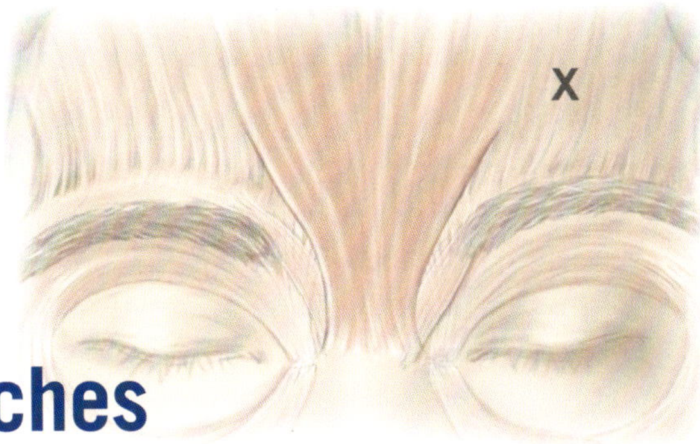

Headaches

Michael S. Benninger

Headaches are one of the most common medical disorders affecting virtually everyone at some point during their lifetime. Tension-type headache (TTH) is the most common type of recurrent primary headache disorder that results in functional limitations.[1,2] The lifetime prevalence of having TTH has been estimated at 30 to as high as 78% of the population.[2] The benefit of botulinum toxin for TTH has been shown in a number of different studies and in controlled trials comparing botulinum toxin to saline injections.[1–3] Of interest, is that the use of botulinum toxin for headaches was somewhat accidental as patients reported headache improvement after undergoing botulinum toxin injection for forehead wrinkles.[4] Studies have also shown effectiveness in the treatment of migraine headaches (MH)[4] although the results have been somewhat less predictable. This in part may be due to the less reliable trigger points where injection seems most effective.

ANATOMIC CONSIDERATIONS

The frontalis muscle, also known as the occipitofrontalis, is a thin muscle that lies over the anterior superior head. Its function is to raise the eyebrows and move the scalp forward and backward. It has its origin from the superior nuchal line of the skull and the mastoid process, as well as the epicranial aponeurosis of the coronal suture. The muscle inserts in the skin of the frontal region, the occipital region, and the galea aponeurosis.[5] The temporalis muscle is a broad, paired fan-shaped muscle on the lateral sides of the head. The function of the temporalis muscle is to elevate the jaw, clench the teeth, and retract the mandible. The muscle originates at the floor of the temporal fossa and in the temporalis fascia. It inserts in the anterior boarder of the ramus and the anterior boarder of the coronoid process of the mandible.[5]

INJECTION TECHNIQUE FOR TENSION-TYPE HEADACHES

The general approach to identifying injection sites for TTH relies on a combination of historical evidence of a trigger point that may be confirmed in most cases through physical examination and palpation. It is not uncommon that 1 or 2 distinct sites can be identified. In our practice the most common trigger sites are in the frontalis (Fig 7–1) or temporalis muscles (Fig 7–2) although it is possible that they will be in the sternocleidomastoid, trapezius, or splenius capitus muscles. There is no fixed appropriate dose and recommendations vary between authors. A reasonable starting point is 5 units of Botox for an identifiable trigger site in the frontalis (see Fig 7–1) or temporalis muscles (see Fig 7–2) and 10 to 15 units in the larger muscles. For diffuse temporalis based head pain, 2 units in 3 or 4 different locations is a reasonable starting point. The dose can be adjusted either up or down based on the response to the initial injection. If there is no identifiable trigger point or area either by history or physical examination then a trial of injections in a manner similar to migraine treatment can

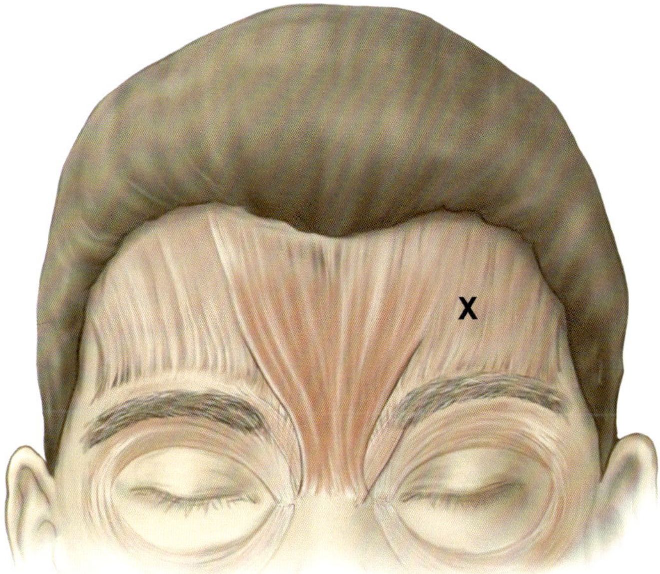

Figure 7–1

be performed. In general, these muscles can be identified without EMG guidance although if EMG is routinely used for injections it does help to verify the location by having the patient flex the associated muscle at the time of injection. Particularly in the glabella and temporal regions and for the larger neck and shoulder muscles, it is reasonable to aspirate the syringe before injection to make sure that the needle is not in the lumen of a vessel.

INJECTION TECHNIQUE FOR MIGRAINE HEADACHES

The location for the injections for migraine have been well described by Binder et al,[4] although other recommendations have been made by other authors. In patients with diffuse

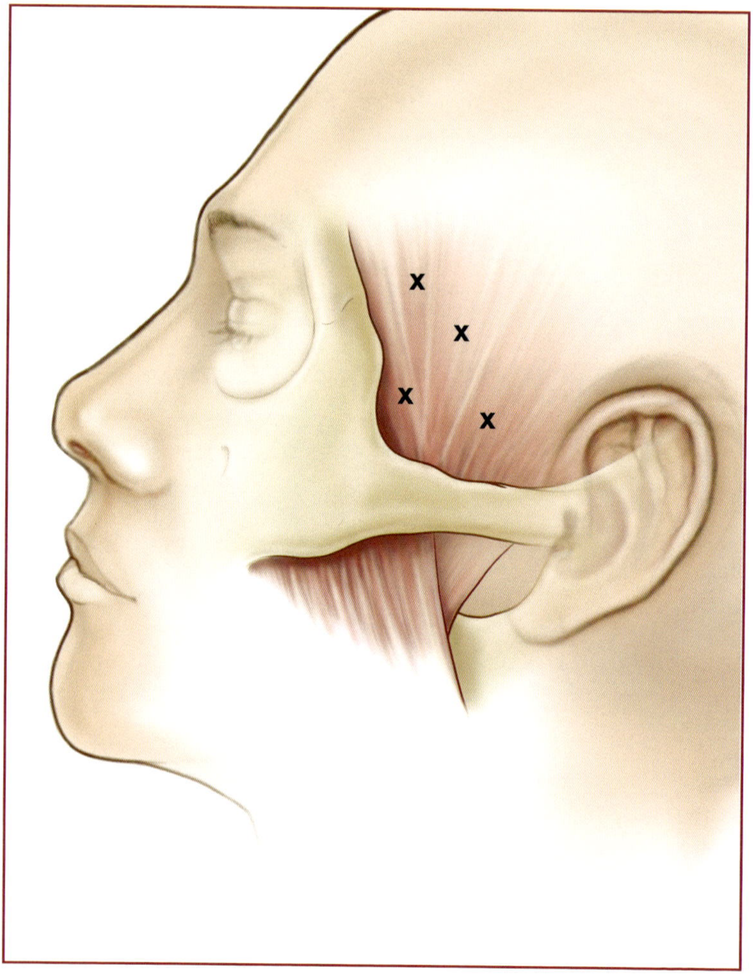

Figure 7–2

migraine headaches, it is more effective to inject multiple sites. A good starting point is to inject 3 forehead, 3 glabella, and 2 temporal sites on each side, and 2 to 3 units per injection site (Fig 7–3). The mean dose of Botox given in the Binder study was 31 units per patient broken up among these sites. Their average number of injection sites per area were 3 to 5 for

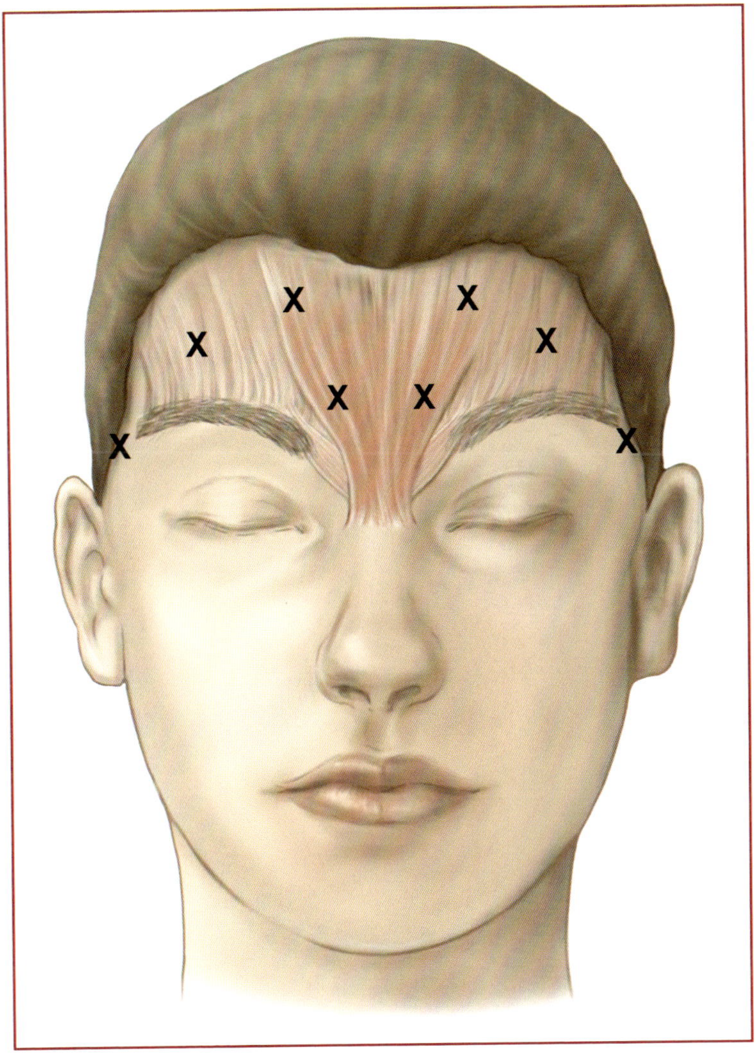

Figure 7–3

glabella, 2 to 4 for each temporal, and 3 to 6 for the forehead. A small minority of patients required additional sub occipital injections but these would not be considered in the standard migraine patient.

REFERENCES

1. Rozen D, Sharma J. Treatment of tension-type headaches with Botox: a review of the literature. *Mt Sinai J Med.* 2006;73:493–498.
2. Hamdy SM, Samir H, El-Sayed M, Adel N, Hasan R. Botulinum toxin: could it be an effective treatment for chronic tension-type headache? *J Headache Pain.* 2008;10:27–34.
3. Porta M. A comparative trial of botulinum toxin A and methylprednisolone for the treatment of tension-type headache. *Curr Rev Pain.* 2000;4:31–35.
4. Binder WJ, Brin MF, Blitzer A, Schoenrock LD, Pogoda JM. Botulinum toxin type A (Botox) for treatment of migraine headaches: an open label study. *Otolaryngol Head Neck Surg.* 2000;123:669–676.
5. Warfel JH. *The Head, Neck and Trunk: Muscles and Motor Points.* 4th ed. Philadelphia, PA: Lea and Febiger; 1978.

CHAPTER

8

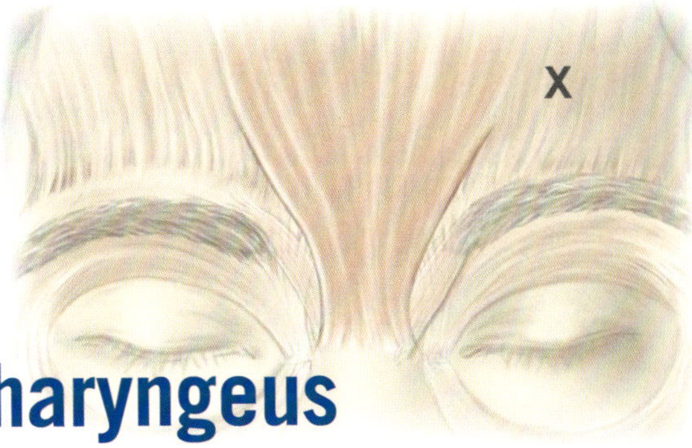

Cricopharyngeus Muscle Dysfunction

Michael S. Benninger

Dysfunction of the cricopharyngeus muscle can be attributed to either functional hyperfunction or mechanical stricture. It is not uncommon in patients who have had a total laryngectomy, particularly if the lower portions of the constrictor muscles or cricopharyngeus are reapproximated at the time of surgery. Cricopharyngeus muscle spasm can be an important cause of dysphagia particularly in the elderly. Botulinum toxin can be an effective treatment for cricopharyngeus muscle hyperfunction or spasm. Botulinum toxin injections for cricopharyngeus dysfunction warrant several considerations. Radiographic evaluation with either a barium esophogram or modified barium swallow should show evidence of contraction of the muscle or a cricopharyngeus bar.

One thing that should be considered before botulinum toxin injection for the cricopharyngeus is the presence of a substantial hiatal hernia or laryngopharyngeal reflux disease. The cricopharyngeus plays an important role in preventing high esophageal reflux from entering the laryngopharynx. Appropriate reflux treatment should be considered in any patient who is planned to undergo botulinum toxin injection for cricopharyngeus dysfunction. In those with poorly controlled reflux, cricopharyngeus treatment should be performed with caution.

ANATOMIC CONSIDERATIONS

The cricopharyngeus is not an independent muscle. Rather, it is the inferior portion of the inferior constrictor muscle. These inferior fibers are horizontal and are continuous with the circular fibers of the esophagus, but because of the thick horizontal muscle bundle they act as a sphincter. These fibers arise from the cricoid cartilage in the interval between the cricothyroideus in front, and the articular facet of the inferior cornua of the thyroid cartilage behind. From these origins the fibers spread backward and medial to insert with the muscle of the opposite side into the pharyngeal raphe in the posterior median line of the pharynx. The muscle's inferior portion lies horizontal to a line extending posteriorly from the lateral aspect of the lower boarder of the cricoid cartilage.[1]

CRICOPHARYNGEUS INJECTION TECHNIQUE

Successful treatment with Botox may require repeat injections as the cricopharyngeus dysfunction returns. On occasion, a patient may get long-term, if not permanent, relief with one or two injections. There are no standard treatment doses for Botox for cricopharyngeus dysfunction and some of the considerations for dosing are the age of the patient, other more substantial swallowing problems, and, as mentioned above, reflux. A good starting dose is 50 to 100 units and this can be done either on one side or bilaterally. We have found that bilateral injections are more effective. In relatively young patients or post laryngectomy, where aspiration is not a concern, 50 units a side is a good starting dose. In older patients or those with other swallowing problems 25 units a side is reasonable. The patients may experience some increased difficulty swallowing for a week or two after the procedure and should be counseled to eat slowly and carefully.

The procedure can be performed in either an upright or reclining position. Locating the cricopharyngeus muscle may be difficult and requires EMG guidance. It can be performed either with or without local anesthesia to the skin over the needle site. The needle is introduced at the midlevel of the cricoid cartilage and is passed laterally hugging the cartilage as closely as possible (Fig 8–1). If the needle is passed too high at the level

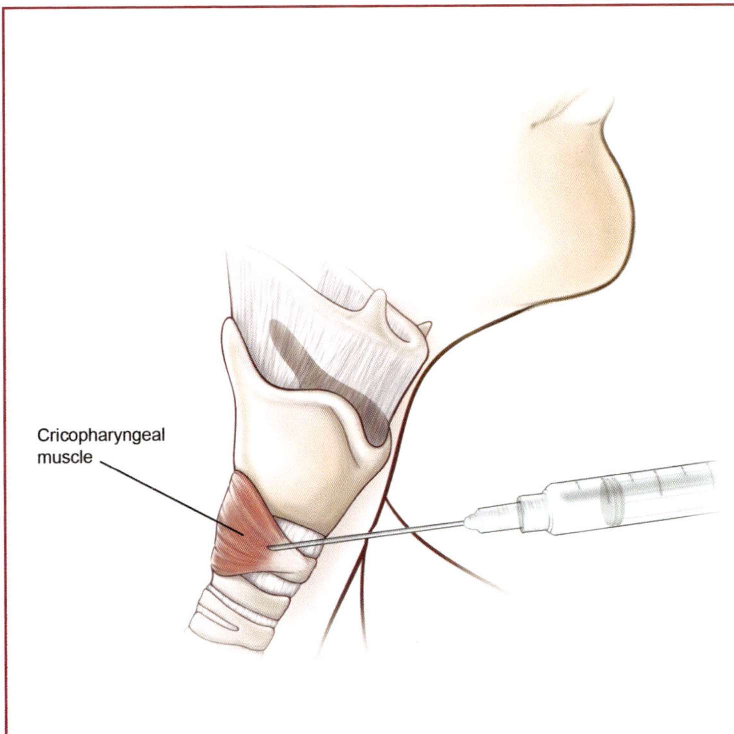

Figure 8–1

of the cricothyroid space, then the needle can enter the cricothyroid muscle. As the cricopharyngeus is contracted at rest, when the needle enters the muscle, tonic EMG activity should be noted. The muscle may be difficult to find and the needle may need to be passed more than once.

The patient is asked to tense their neck muscles to ensure that the needle is not in a strap muscle, where increased activity would occur. A simple way to contract the neck strap muscles without moving the neck is to have the patient clench their teeth. Once it is felt that the needle is in the cricopharyngeus, it can be confirmed by having the patient swallow. If in the correct spot, there should be a decrease in activity followed by return of EMG signal. In some people there may be a short increase in EMG signal just prior to the decrease, and then a return to normal chronic muscle activity. On occasion, the needle may slip from the muscle with the movement of the swallow and the EMG signal may be lost. It is usually easier to find the muscle the second time. The needle should be aspirated to assure that an intravascular injection will not occur and 25 to 50 units of Botox are injected. The volume of the Botox mix should be small enough that it will not cause much discomfort or disperse into the surrounding neck muscles, but large enough to reach multiple muscle fibers in the cricopharyngeus; 0.5 to 1 mL per side is reasonable. The same technique is then used to inject the other side.

CRICOPHARYNGEUS INJECTION FOLLOWING TOTAL LARYNGECTOMY

Cricopharyngeus dysfunction is not uncommon following total laryngectomy and Botox serves as an excellent first option. This is particularly true as surgical management of persistent cricopharyngeus muscle contraction in patients who already have had neck surgery and often have also had radiation or combined chemotherapy with radiation. The concerns related to reflux aspiration are not a concern.

As the location of the cricopharyngeus or upper esophageal sphincter areas may have been altered by the surgery, locating the muscle may be difficult and require multiple needle passes, so it is not unreasonable to inject the skin of the injection site. The cricopharyngeus usually sits above the stoma site and a good first place to pass the needle is at a line drawn horizontally from the upper edge of the stoma and one drawn superiorly and vertically from the most lateral aspect of the stoma (Fig 8–2). The needle is entered until tonic muscle contraction is identified. Verification of the location is done the

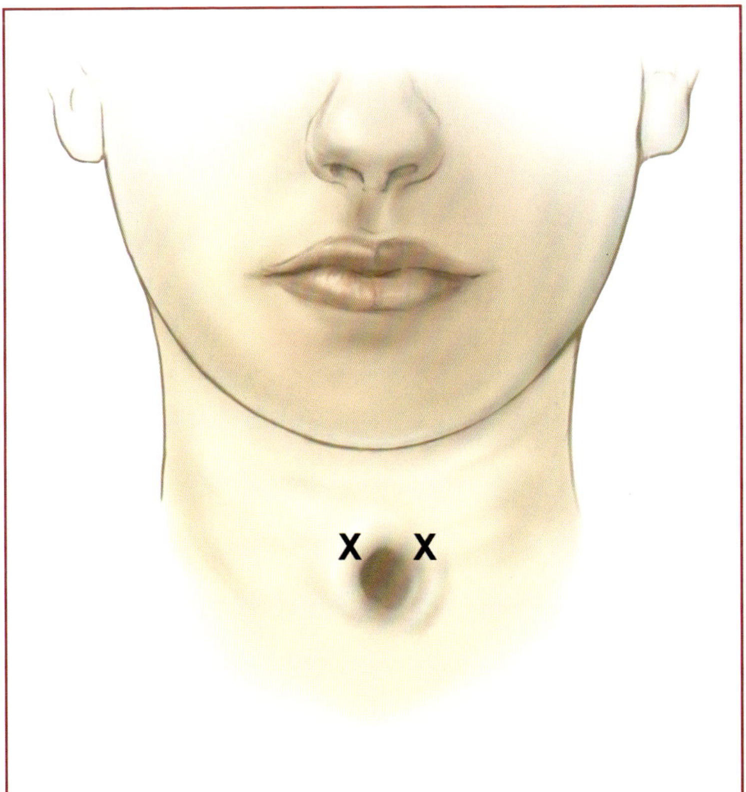

Figure 8–2

same way as when a patient has an intact larynx. The patient is asked to tense their neck muscles to ensure that the needle is not in a strap muscle, where increased activity would occur. Once it is felt that the needle is in the cricopharyngeus, the patient can then swallow and the location is confirmed. The needle is aspirated and the injection can be made. As there is not the same concern of aspiration as with an intact larynx, we usually inject 50 units of Botox per side.

REFERENCE

1. Warfel JH. *The Head, Neck and Trunk: Muscles and Motor Points*. 4th ed. Philadelphia, PA: Lea and Febiger; 1978.

CHAPTER

9

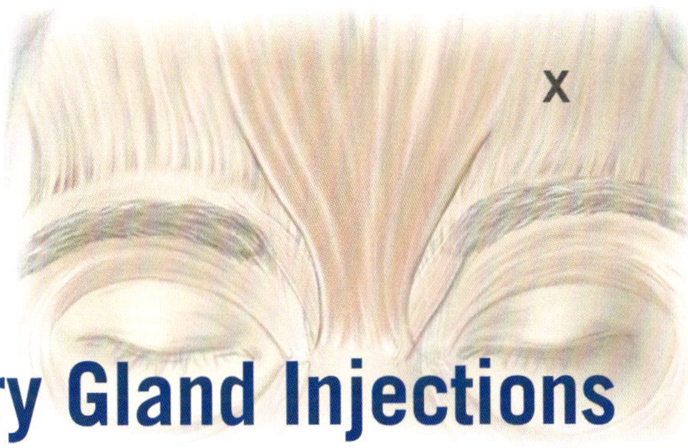

Salivary Gland Injections

Michael S. Benninger

Salivary gland disorders with chronic sialorrhea can be very disturbing to both patients and their families. Poorly controlled sialorrhea usually occurs in neurologically impaired children or adults and is a common feature in many progressive neurologic degenerative diseases such as amyotrophic lateral sclerosis, but it also common in focal neurological disorders such as Bell's palsy. In children it can be seen in mental retardation and cerebral palsy as well as other disorders. Sialorrhia can be defined as: "involuntary, passive pooling and spillage of saliva from the mouth due to inability to process oral secretions."[1] It has been estimated that each adult individual produces up to a liter of saliva a day with 90% of this being produced through the parotid and submandibular glands.[2] Although there is pharmacological treatment that is effective in partial management of the sialorrhea, many patients continue to have persistent difficulties with drooling or do not tolerate the side effects of the medications, particularly with systemic anticholinergics or sedating antihistamines. In such cases botulinum toxin has been shown to be an effective and relatively simple treatment option.[1,3,4]

ANATOMIC CONSIDERATIONS

The saliva glands are exocrine glands with ducts that produce a number of substances, principally saliva and amylase. There are 3 paired major salivary glands and numerous small minor salivary glands. The parotid glands are the largest of the major salivary glands and sit lateral to mandibular ramus and the masseter muscles. There is a component that lies in the posterior neck beneath the ear lobule. The secretions are mainly serous and are excreted via Stenson's duct behind the 2nd maxillary molar. The submandibular glands are in the upper neck beneath the mandible and superior to the digastric muscles. The secretions are a mix of serous and mucous and enter the mouth through Wharton's ducts in the floor of the mouth.

Although 60 to 70% of saliva is produced from the submandibular glands, the more dependent flow of the saliva posteriorly along the floor of the mouth allows for a more ready clearance and may account for why parotid gland injections alone can provide relief of sialorrhea, particularly in adults. The more neurologically compromised a patient is, the more likely that submandibular gland secretions need to be managed.

INJECTION TECHNIQUES

The dose of Botox treatment varies between studies and in adults versus children, and many authors advocate different dosing regimens. Most authors recommend 3 separate injection sites per gland. In adults we routinely use 10 units in 3 individual sites (Fig 9–1) in each parotid gland, constituted to have 30 units in 0.9 mL of 0.9% sodium chloride. Larger volumes are associated with more discomfort. In general, we do not use local anesthesia as the discomfort of the anesthesia is equal to or greater than that of the 25- or 27-gauge needle used for injection. In general we start with parotid gland injections and then

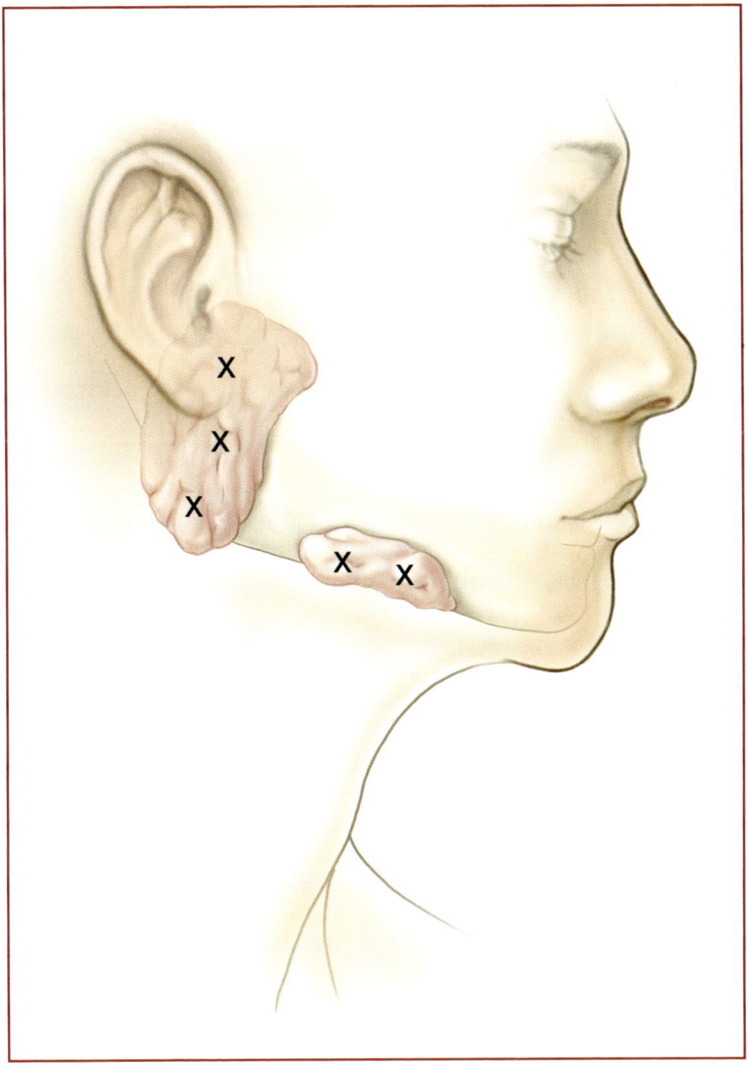

Figure 9–1

proceed to submandibular gland injections at a different setting based on the response to the parotid injections. A similar dose of Botox of 30 units per gland is used in the submandibular gland. EMG can be used to assist, but because the injections are into the gland and not the muscle, EMG is helpful only to suggest where not to inject.

In children the dose can be formulated to give 5 units/kg divided among the injected glands; or 15 units per gland for children under 15 kg, 20 units per gland for children 15 to 25 kg, and 25 units per gland for children 25 kg or more.[3] In the latter dosing as advocated by Scheffer,[3] only the submandibular glands were injected.

REFERENCES

1. Khan WU, Campisi P, Nadarajah S, et al. Boltulinum toxin A for the treatment of sialorrhea in children: An effective, minimally invasive approach. *Arch Otolaryngol Head Neck Surg.* 2011; Published online Jan 17 (doi:10.1001/archoto.2010.240).
2. Hockstein NG, Samadi DS, Gendron K, et al. Sialorrhea: a management challege. *Am Fam Physician.* 2004;69:2628–2634.
3. Scheffer ART, Erasmus C, van Hulst K, et al. Efficacy and duration of botulinum toxin treatment for drooling in 131 children. *Arch Otolaryngol Head Neck Surg.* 2010;136:873–877.
4. Raval TH, Elliott CA. Botulinum toxin injection to the salivary glands for the treatment of sialorrhea with chronic aspiration. *Ann Otol Rhinol Laryngol.* 2008;117:118–122.

CHAPTER

10

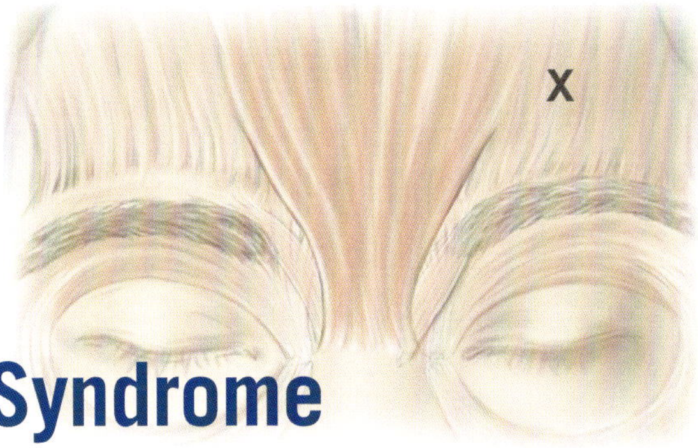

Frey's Syndrome

Peter C. Revenaugh

Frey's syndrome, also known as gustatory sweating, commonly occurs following parotid surgery. The syndrome is characterized by flushing and hyperhidrosis of the cheek and preauricular skin during mastication. Reported symptoms include sweating, flushing, and sensations of warmth, tingling, swelling, and/or itching.[1] Patients report discomfort and embarrassment when eating which negatively impacts quality of life.[2]

In 1923, a Polish neurologist, Lucie Frey, postulated a relationship between the auriculotemporal nerve and gustatory sweating in a patient who had been slashed with a knife.[3] Several years later, Thomas proposed the aberrant regeneration theory that is the basis of our current understanding of the pathophysiology of the syndrome.[4] The aberrant regeneration theory postulates that parasympathetic fibers traveling from the otic ganglion to the salivary glandular tissue are damaged through trauma. These cut cholinergic parasympathetic fibers are then misdirected during regeneration to innervate cholinergic sympathetic receptors of the subcutaneous vessels and sweat glands.

Parotidectomy is the leading cause of gustatory sweating; 10 to 40% of patients note or complain of gustatory sweating following parotidectomy.[5] However, by using Minor's starch iodine test where starch is applied to the cheek followed by ingestion of a sialogogue, upward of 95% of postparotidectomy patients are affected by the syndrome.[6]

Topical anticholinergic medications, such as scopolamine and glycopyrrolate, can be effective but require reapplication, carry several side effects such as dry mouth, and caution must be observed in patients with glaucoma.[5] Within the last 15 years, botulinum toxin has been described as a promising new treatment. Drobik and colleagues reported the first use of botulinum toxin for the treatment of Frey's syndrome in 1995.[7] Almost complete resolution of gustatory sweating was observed in their report. Since that time, several large studies have been conducted (Table 10–1). The period of effective treatment observed for Frey's syndrome averages 17.3 months, which is longer than that observed for other head and neck applications treating neuromuscular sites.[8]

ANATOMIC CONSIDERATIONS

The parotid is the largest of the salivary glands, with a mean dimension of 5.8 by 3.4 cm and a mean weight of 14 grams. It lies within the parotid compartment, which also contains the facial nerve, sensory and autonomic nerves, and the terminal external branch of the carotid artery, parotid lymphatics, and the posterior facial vein. It overlies the masseter and mandible, and a portion extends over the superior quarter of the sternocleidomastoid muscle inferior to the lobule of the ear and extends in some cases to the mastoid process.

Table 10–1. *Studies Reporting Botox Treatment*

Study	Year of Publication	Number of Patients	Follow-Up (months)	Dose	Recurrence (%)
Naumann et al[9]	1997	45	6	21 MU*	0.0
Laskawi et al[8]	1998	18	11 to 33	31.3 U*	44.0
Laccourreye et al[12]	1999	33	>18	86 U*	92.0
Eckardt et al[1]	2003	33	6 to 18	16 to 80 U	27.6
Kyrmizakis et al[10]	2004	11	6 to 23	25 U*	9.0

MU = mouse-units; U = units; * = denotes mean value.

INJECTION TECHNIQUE

Botox treatment of gustatory sweating is easily performed in an outpatient setting. The exact area of treatment may be determined via Minor's starch iodine test or may be observed directly as a moist area surrounded by flushing following gustatory stimulation (eating). A typical area of treatment averages approximately 20 to 30 cm^2. There are several simple, yet important, principles to consider with this treatment. Each injection should be made in the intradermal plane, in order to correctly target the sweat glands and dermal and subdermal vascularity. Furthermore, the injections should only be performed in the area which bothers the patient, typically in the preauricular and infralobular skin above and behind the angle of the mandible (Fig 10–1). Although any dilution of botulinum toxin may be used, typically less concentrated treatment is favored. After the affected area is divided into square centimeter units, intradermal injection of Botox is completed. Doses vary between 0.5 U/cm^2 and 2U/2.25 cm^2.[1,7,9,10] Total doses range from 20 to 80 units, although we usually favor 20 to 30 units. Following treatment, gustatory sweating usually ceases within 2 days.

Caution must be used to not inject deeper than the intradermal plane and not beyond 2 to 3 cm anterior to the tragus, in order to avoid inadvertent treatment of the muscles of facial expression.[11] Recurrent symtpomatic sweating, if it occurs, is typically less severe and responds well to retreatment.

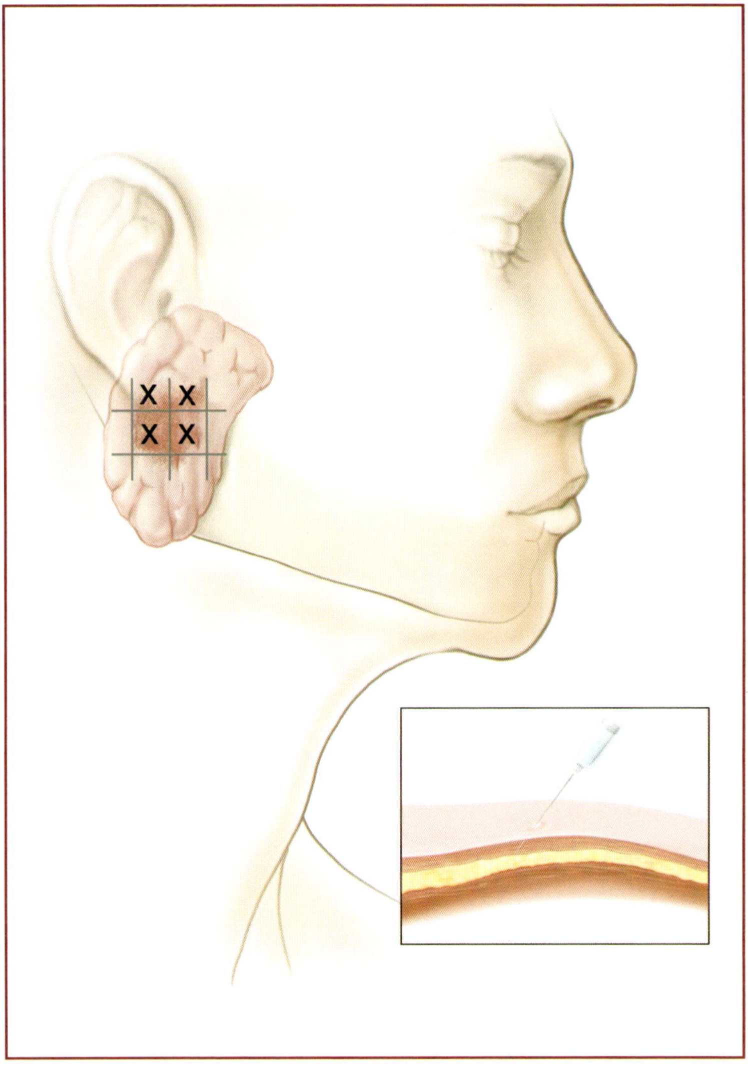

Figure 10–1

REFERENCES

1. Eckardt A, Kuettner C. Treatment of gustatory sweating (Frey's syndrome) with botulinum toxin A. *Head Neck.* Aug 2003;25(8):624–628.
2. Nitzan D, Kronenberg J, Horowitz Z, et al. Quality of life following parotidectomy for malignant and benign disease. *Plast Reconstr Surg.* Oct 2004;114(5):1060–1067.
3. Frey L. Le syndrome du nerf auriculo-temporal. *Rev Neurol.* 1923;2: 97–104.
4. Thomas A. Le double reflexe vaso-dilatateur et sudoral de la face consecutive aux blessures de la loge parotidienne. *Rev Neurol (Paris).* 1927;1:447–460.
5. de Bree R, van der Waal I, Leemans CR. Management of Frey syndrome. *Head Neck.* Aug 2007;29(8):773–778.
6. Linder TE, Huber A, Schmid S. Frey's syndrome after parotidectomy: a retrospective and prospective analysis. *Laryngoscope.* Nov 1997;107 (11 pt 1):1496–1501.
7. Drobik C, Laskawi R. Frey's syndrome: treatment with botulinum toxin. *Acta Otolaryngol.* May 1995;115(3):459–461.
8. Laskawi R, Drobik C, Schonebeck C. Up-to-date report of botulinum toxin type A treatment in patients with gustatory sweating (Frey's syndrome). *Laryngoscope.* Mar 1998;108(3):381–384.
9. Naumann M, Zellner M, Toyka KV, Reiners K. Treatment of gustatory sweating with botulinum toxin. *Ann Neurol.* Dec 1997;42(6):973–975.
10. Kyrmizakis DE, Pangalos A, Papadakis CE, Logothetis J, Maroudias NJ, Helidonis ES. The use of botulinum toxin type A in the treatment of Frey and crocodile tears syndromes. *J Oral Maxillofac Surg.* Jul 2004; 62(7):840–844.
11. Laskawi R, Rohrbach S. Treatment of gustatory sweating with botulinum toxin: special aspects. *ORL J Otorhinolaryngol Relat Spec.* 2001 Sep–Oct;63(5):294–297.
12. Laccourreye O, Akl E, Gutierrez-Fonseca R, et al. Recurrent sweating (Frey syndrome) after intracutaneous injection of botulinum toxin type A: incidence, management, and outcome. *Arch Otolaryngol Head Neck Surg.* Mar 1990;125(3)283–286.

SECTION

III

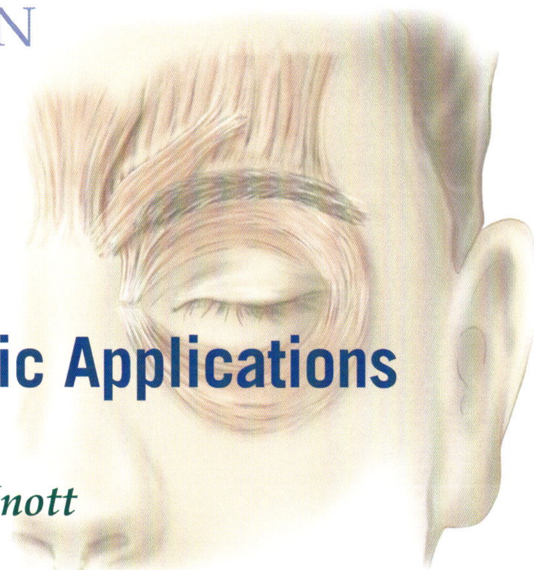

Cosmetic Applications

P. Daniel Knott

Treatment of the aging face in recent decades has become both more sophisticated and more simple. The sophistication lies in the myriad of treatment options available to the rejuvenative practitioner: multiple injectable volumizers, laser resurfacing, chemical peels, implants and suspension devices, structural fat grafting, skin-tightening technologies, and a variety of face-lifting techniques, to name just a few. The simplicity presents in the relative ease of use and public embrace of botulinum toxin, such that a new population of providers is both eager and capable of providing effective treatment.

Botulinum toxin is a very useful adjunct to any rejuvenative approach for patients in their thirties or eighties. It is commonly understood that treatment of the aging face must address four major conditions: soft tissue descent, photoaging, soft tissue atrophy, and the formation of dynamic rhytids. Of these categories, treatment of dynamic wrinkles with botulinum toxin is the most straightforward, the most effective, and has the least downtime. Therefore, any practitioner with an interest in offering rejuvenative services needs to develop skills in the application of botulinum toxin.

Once simply called "botox," botulinum toxin has evolved into a pharmaceutical goliath, with many companies competing for this lucrative market. Allergan markets Botox Cosmetic and Medicis markets Dysport. Another formulation called Xeomin will be released imminently, and yet another topically-applied form of botulinum toxin will likely be released soon. Another subtype of botulinum toxin, type B, is marketed as Myobloc.

Despite the rapidly expanding product line for botulinum toxin, gaining facility and confidence with one formulation is recommended. Excellent, reliable, and reproducible results depend on attention to detail with accurate dilutions, the delivery of precise unit volumes, and fine anatomic understanding. This section will help establish an effective and safe practice in facial rejuvenation.

CHAPTER

11

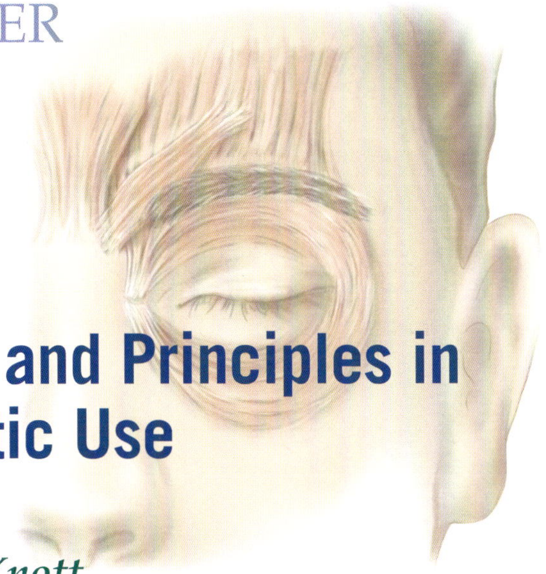

Theory and Principles in Aesthetic Use

P. Daniel Knott

The aesthetic use of botulinum toxin has literally changed the face of the aesthetic treatment of premature aging and head and neck paralytic disorders. When used in appropriate doses and in the appropriate areas, botulinum toxin represents an extremely powerful tool for softening or eliminating wrinkles and hyperdynamic lines (rhytids), balancing eyebrows, and restoring facial symmetry both at rest and with animation. From the perspective of a facial plastic surgeon, botulinum toxin stands in a class of its own, and forms an important component of any comprehensive rejuvenative strategy. One must simply remember to determine the cause of the wrinkles, as lines caused by sun exposure, smoking, or gravity-induced sagging usually will not be significantly improved with the injection of botulinum toxin.

Facial movement and expressiveness results from the complicated concert of interactive facial muscles. With 20 paired muscles on each facial half, facial expression is the manifestation of a fabulous diversity of potential muscle interaction. Due to its potential to partially or completely chemodenervate single muscles or entire muscle groups, botulinum toxin has the potential to dramatically alter or enhance facial expressiveness. Prior to initiating a treatment, a firm understanding of the potency, potential for diffusion, and depth of target tissue of botulinum toxin must be developed, not to mention a close study of individual patients and their particular patterns of emotiveness and anatomical variants. Usually, botulinum toxin is administered equally to both facial halves when used for aesthetic purposes, but occasionally unequal fractions are injected to correct subtle asymmetries. Therefore, a detailed discussion must occur during the first consultation in order to gain an understanding of the patients' motivations and perspectives, and to develop an appropriate and effective treatment protocol. As botulinum effectiveness persists for 3 to 6 months, a pleased patient will usually return for future treatments.

Dynamic facial wrinkles result from the repetitive contraction and relaxation of underlying muscles of facial expression, which are arranged perpendicular to the orientation of the overlying rhytid. These muscles begin functioning in earnest in infancy and continue throughout life, with the only exception occurring in patients suffering from facial paralysis. The continual, repetitive contraction and relaxation of these muscles, occurring hundreds to thousands of times per day, inexorably etches wrinkles into the face, just as the continual flow of water and blowing of wind carves notches and digs canyons into cliff faces and valley floors.

Each individual develops his or her individual facial signature over time, depending on his or her particular pattern of repetitive facial movement. This phenomenon may be seen among the older generation, whose distinctive pattern is well established with a dominant expression visible at rest. This is the end result of lifelong repetitive emotional expressiveness. The particular severity and pattern of wrinkle formation follows several principles. The first principle is that rhytid potential is related to the distance between the skin and the muscle and the degree with which the two are joined by connective tissue, that is, the more superficial the muscle the greater is its potential for creating facial rhytids. The second principle is that rhytid development is directly related to the frequency of use and strength of each particular muscle.

When muscles act alone without opposing forces, the use of a neuroparalytic agent such as botulinum toxin, causes a flaccid paralysis and softening or obliteration of the overlying wrinkles, as in the case of the glabella and the lateral crow's feet. When used in an area characterized by competing muscle vectors, such as in the brow or perioral region, the botulinum toxin weakens or paralyzes one muscle group, thereby tilting the balance to the competing muscle(s), and shifting the overlying skin and cutaneous structures. Therefore, the competitive interaction of muscle groups must be understood, such that the balance is tilted in a deliberate and desired fashion.

AGENTS AND CONCENTRATIONS

There are two popular, commercially available preparations of botulinum toxin A, which dominate the marketplace. Botox Cosmetic (Onabotulinum toxin A, Allergan Pharmaceuticals, Irvine CA) and Dysport (Abobotulinum toxin A, Medicis Pharmaceutical, Scottsdale AZ). Other formulations include Myobloc, Xeomin, Neurobloc, and Neuronox. Botox Cosmetic was the first to receive FDA approval for aesthetic use in the glabella in 2002, with Dysport following in 2009. Comparison studies of these two, dominant products demonstrate approximately equivalent effectiveness, average onset, and duration of action, although Dysport may have a tendency toward greater diffusion and shorter duration of effect at a dose ratio of 2.5:1 (Dysport:Botox Cosmetic).[1] Cosmetic use of botulinum toxin is not recommended among patients with egg allergies or neuromuscular disorders, or among pregnant or lactating females.

No deaths have ever been ascribed to cosmetic use of botulinum toxin. Particular safety profiles and contraindications should be reviewed on the package inserts or on the producer's Web sites.

INJECTION TECHNIQUE

Botulinum toxin may be injected in intramuscular, subcutaneous, or dermal planes. The depth of the injection depends on the depth of the target muscle, and the concentration of the solution. Bleeding is rarely encountered, even with intramuscular depositions, and is best treated with a brief application of firm manual pressure. Concomitant use of anti-coagulants, such as warfarin, aspirin, and Plavix is not specifically contraindicated, although caution is recommended. Photodocumentation should be performed before every injection, and the amount and location of each injection should be recorded. Topical anesthetics and nerve blocks are usually not required. Doses and injection sites will vary between patients and the recommendations enumerated in this text should serve as a starting point for an individualized treatment plan and providers should always adhere to the maxim, "as much as necessary and as little as possible."

BOTOX COSMETIC

Botox Cosmetic is prepared as a dehydrated purified form of toxin and is packaged in a vacuum-sealed 100 unit vial. Reconstitution is recommended with sterile, preservative-free 0.9% saline. Gentle swirling of the bottle creates a smooth and even concentration. The manufacturer recommends discarding the unused component after 4 hours, although studies have shown maintenance of efficacy for up to 6 weeks following reconstitution, if stored at a temperature of 2 to 8 degrees Celsius.[2]

The concentration of Botox Cosmetic will vary depending on the volume of saline used for reconstitution. This is a key concept. Dosing for facial aesthetic purposes differs dramatically from other functional uses. Recommendations for the volume of saline used for reconstitution vary from 1 to 4 mLs.[3–6] The use of larger volumes of saline for reconstitution (lower concentration) means that higher volumes will be required to deliver the desired number of units of the toxin, with the potential for increased diffusion. Lower volumes of reconstitution (higher concentration) means lower volumes will be required for injection, with likely decreased potential for diffusion. With higher concentrations, greater precision of the injection is necessary. Furthermore, the use of higher volumes for reconstitution adds complexity to tallying the amount of the toxin injected, particularly when doing multiple injections in multiple subsites while maintaining adherence to precise bilaterality of the injection, as is usually the case.

A very useful reconstitution will be achieved with 1 mL of saline per vial, such that each 0.01-mL notch on the syringe corresponds to 1 unit of Botox Cosmetic. Epinephrine may be added to further restrict diffusion, but this is not routinely performed. When aspirating the final 10 units from each bottle, I recommend removing the bottle top and aspirating the remaining solution directly from the bottom of the bottle. When treating the frontalis, a lower concentration may be advantageous, as it allows similar efficacy using fewer units and diffusion of the toxin may be advantageous.

I recommend the use of 0.3 mL Ultra-Fine insulin syringes with the attached 30-g, 8-mm needle. These latex-free, single-use syringes (BD, Becton, Dickinson and Company) are small and greatly simplify the process of injection. With the above mentioned reconstitution formula, each syringe contains a maximum of 30 units of Botox Cosmetic, and therefore multiple syringes may be required. Depending on the number of subsites addressed, I prefer to use 1 syringe per facial half, or 1 syringe per subsite. When injecting multiple subsites, the need to use multiple syringes ensures that the needle stays sharp and pain is minimized.

DYSPORT

Dysport is supplied as a single-use, sterile, 300 unit non-vacuum-sealed vial, which is likewise reconstituted with sterile, preservative-free, 0.9% sodium chloride solution. Just as with Botox Cosmetic, Dysport may be reconstituted with different volumes of saline, yielding different ultimate concentrations. Once again, I recommend developing a system of optimal concentration in order to simplify the injection process and minimize the potential for diffusion. The approximate clinical efficacy correlation between Botox Cosmetic and Dysport is 1:2 to 1:4.[7] Therefore, for the approximate similar clinical effect, 2 to 4 times as many units of Dysport need to be injected for each unit of botox that is usually injected. I recommend reconstitution with 1.5 mL of saline for the Dysport, yielding a concentration of 2 units/0.01 mL. Using a correlation factor of approximately 1:2 (Botox Cosmetic:Dysport), 0.01 mL of Dysport needs to be injected for each 0.01 mL of Botox Cosmetic.

For the remainder of Section III, I recommend unit doses of Botox Cosmetic, and highlight the units of Dysport in parentheses.

REFERENCES

1. Lowe PI, Patnaik R, Lowe NJ. A comparison of two botulinum type A toxin preparations for the treatment of glabellar lines: double-blind, randomized, pilot study. *Dermatol Surg*. 2005;31:1651.
2. Hexsel D, De Almeida AT, Rutowotsch M, et al. Multicenter double blind study of the efficacy of injections with botulinum toxin type A

reconstituted up to six consecutive weeks before application. *Dermatol Surg*. 2003;29:523–529.
3. Blitzer A, Brin MF, Keen MF, et al. Botulinum toxin for the treatment of hyperfunctional lines of the face. *Arch Otolaryngol Head Neck Surg*. 1993;119:1018–1022.
4. Carruthers JDA, Gloglau RG, Blitzer A, et al. Advances in facial rejuvenation: botulinum toxin type A, hyaluronic acid dermal fillers, and combination therapies-consensus recommendations. *Plast Reconstr Surg*. 2008;121:5–30S.
5. Kane M, Donofrio L, Ascher B, et al. Expanding the use of neurotoxins in facial aesthetics: a consensus panel's assessment and recommendations. *J Drugs Dermatol*. 2010;9:S7–22.
6. Baumann L, Brandt FS, Kane MA, et al. An analysis of efficacy data from four phase III studies of botulinum neurotoxin type A-ABO for the treatment of glabellar lines. *Aesthet Surg J*. 2009;29:S57–65.
7. Karsai S, Raulin C. Botox and Dysport: is there a dose conversion ratio in dermatology and aesthetic medicine? *J Am Acad Dermatol*. 2010;62(2):346–347.

CHAPTER

12

Glabella

P. Daniel Knott

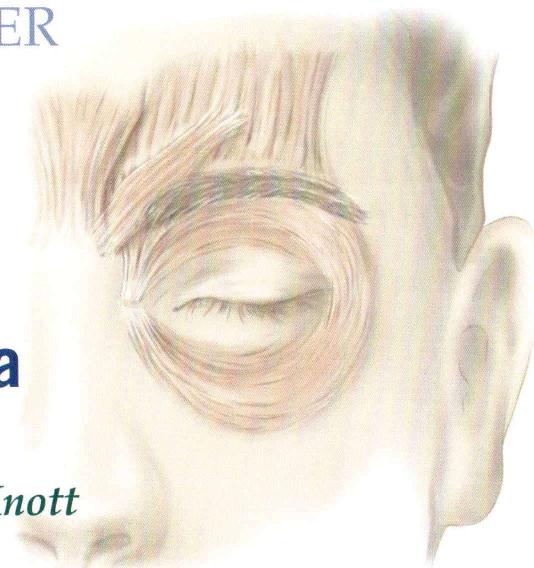

The glabella is one of the most important and earliest facial regions that may benefit from treatment with botulinum toxin. Located at the center of the brows and directly over the nose, the glabella is characterized by intersections of multiple muscles at differing depths and different relative strengths. The muscles at the glabella coordinate to produce squinting, frowning, and medial brow elevation with expressions of surprise, anger, and dismay. The expressions generated from muscle contraction at the glabella are generally negative, and therefore this subsite may be treated relatively aggressively. If patients want to maintain some degree of expressiveness at the glabella, initial treatment should be conservative, with follow-up injections 1 to 2 weeks later as needed for persistent muscle action.

ANATOMIC CONSIDERATIONS

Corrugator Supercilli

The corrugator is an obliquely oriented muscle that originates on the frontal bone centrally and then travels in a deep to superficial manner, interdigitating with the frontalis, before inserting into the skin of the forehead approximately 1 to 2 centimeters above the mid-brow (Fig 12–1). With contraction, this muscle pulls the medial brow centrally and inferiorly, causing the vertically oriented glabellar wrinkle.

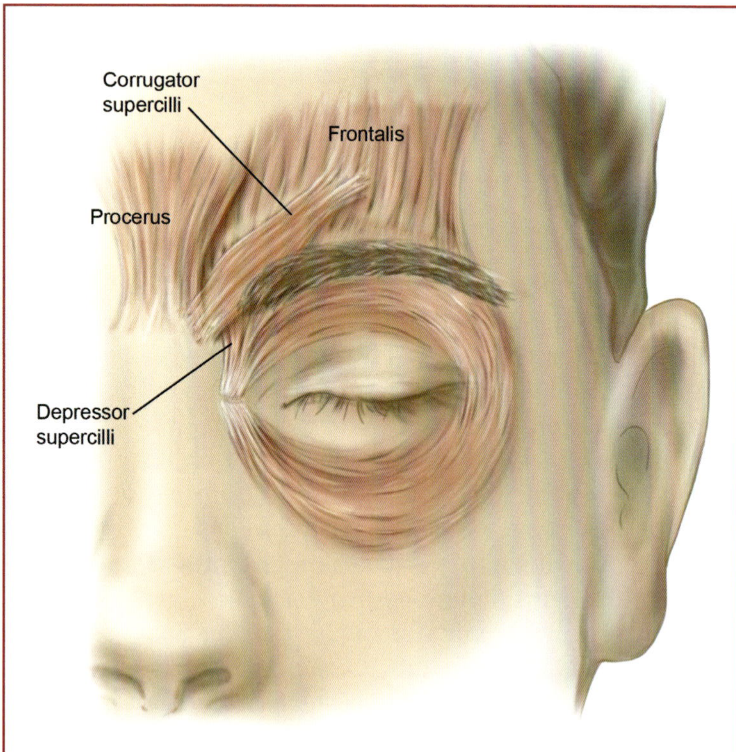

Figure 12–1

Depressor Supercilii

The depressor originates from the frontal process of the maxilla approximately 1 cm above the medial canthus and inserts into the dermis near the medial head of the eyebrow (see Fig 12–1). Its contraction pulls the medial brow in a more inferior vector than the corrugator supercilli.

Procerus

The procerus muscle is an unpaired, central muscle that originates off of the nasal bones and inserts into the dermis in the midline of the glabella, after interdigitating with the corrugator (see Fig 12–1). With contraction, the procerus causes the horizontal wrinkles at the top of the nose between the eyes (aka bunny lines).

Frontalis

The frontalis muscles are the only brow elevators. These large, flat, and wide muscles originate from the galea aponeurotica at or above the hairline, and insert into the dermis at or above the brows, after interdigitating with the fibers of the procerus and corrugator (see Fig 12–1). With contraction, the frontalis muscles raise the brows and cause the horizontal wrinkles that extend across the forehead.

INJECTION TECHNIQUE

The corrugator may be treated with 2 to 3 injections per side using 12–15 units of Botox Cosmetic (24–30 units of Dysport) (Fig 12–2).[1–4] With the first treatment, a conservative to intermediate dose is recommended. If the patient does not gain

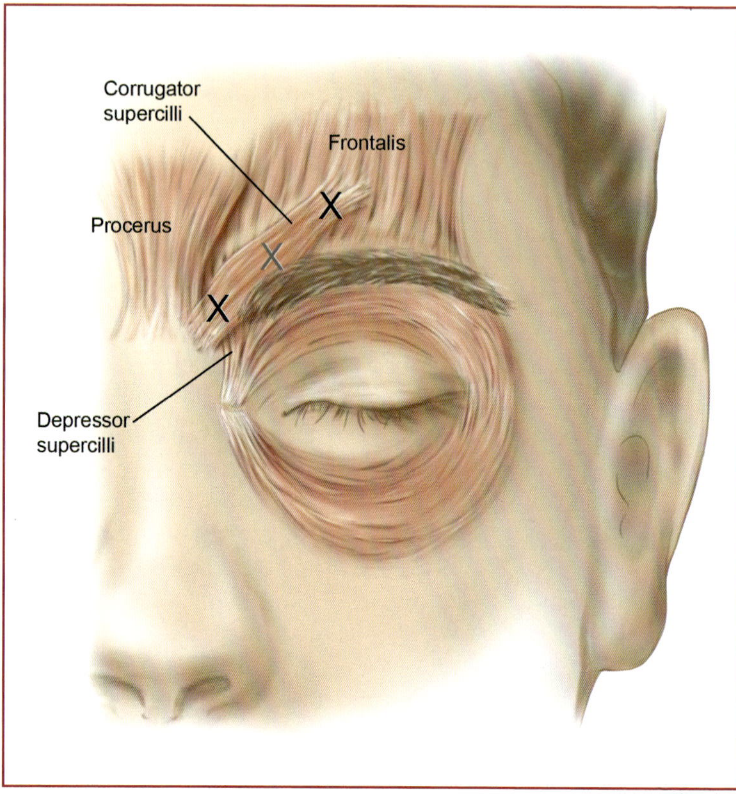

Figure 12–2

satisfactory results after 7 days, then a repeat "booster" injection may be performed. After asking the patient to "frown," the first injection is performed approximately 1 cm lateral to the midline, usually near the largest visible rhytid. The needle is inserted until gentle bone contact is made. It is then slightly withdrawn and and half of the chosen dose of botulinum toxin is delivered intramuscularly. The patient is then asked to frown a second time and the insertion of the muscle into the dermis above the midbrow is noted, where a furrow is created when the skin is pulled inferomedially. At a point at least 1 cm above the level of the native brow, the second injection is made quite superficially, into the dermis and immediate subdermis. If the injection is precise and only the corrugator is targeted, the medial brow will rise modestly, giving the patient a more awake and refreshed look.

Caution: If the second injection above the brow is performed too deeply, or if the medial injection is performed too superfically, the frontalis muscle will also be treated and will subsequently lose function. This may lead to a depression of the medial brow. This may be balanced by the mild elevation that occurs with the treatment of the corrugator, but should be avoided, as it may result in a slightly "angry" appearance.

Additionally, the importance of the injection being performed at least 1 centimeter above the medial brow needs to be stressed. The botulinum, even in the recommended concentrated doses, will partially diffuse through the tissues. If injected at or below the level of the brow, the botulinum may diffuse unimpeded directly to the eyelid elevators and cause resulting temporary dysfunction and depression of the eyelid (blepharoptosis or half-lidded expression) in up to 3.2% of treatments.[5] Although eventually reversible over several months as the botulinum effect wanes, this complication will lead to an extremely dissatisfied patient. In this situation, sympathomimetic eyedrops can ameliorate the unwanted effect. I recommend apraclonidine 0.5% into the affected eye 2 to 3 times daily. This may raise the eyelid several millimeters and restore symmetry.

For the procerus I recommend a single injection site in the midline using 6 to 8 units of Botox Cosmetic (12–16 units of Dysport) (Fig 12–3). I ask the patient to "squinch your nose" to localize the center of the muscle. Then, I inject in a subdermal plane centrally. Then partially withdraw your needle and reinject in both lateral directions in the same plane along the sidewalls of the nose. In this fashion, the complete muscle may be treated with one needle insertion.

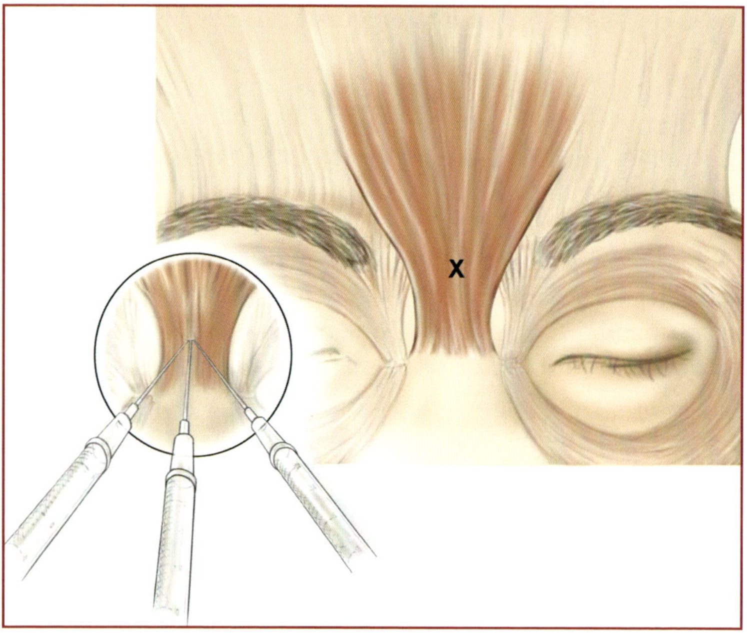

Figure 12–3

REFERENCES

1. Monheit G, Carruthers A, Brandt F, Rand R. A randomized, double-blind, placebo-controlled study of botulinum toxin type A for the treatment of glabellar lines: determination of optimal dose. *Dermatol Surg*. 2007;33(1);S51–59.
2. Kane MA, Brandt F, Rohrich RJ, et al. Evaluation of variable-dose treatment with a new US botulinum toxin type A (Dysport) for correction of moderate to severe glabellar lines: results from a phase III, randomized, double-blind, placebo-controlled study. *Plast Reconstr Surg*. 2009:124(5)1619–1629.
3. Rzany B, Ascher B, Fratila A, et al. Efficacy and safety of 3- and 5-injection patterns (30 and 50 U) of botulinum toxin A (Dysport) for the treatment of wrinkles in the glabella and the central forehead region. *Arch Dermatol*. 2006;142(3):320–326.

4. Blitzer A, Binder WJ, Aviv JE, Keen MS, Brin MF. The management of hyperfunctional facial lines with botulinum toxin. A collaborative study of 210 injection sites in 162 patients. *Arch Otolaryngol Head Neck Surg.* 1997;123(4):389–392.
5. Framptom JE, Easthope SE. Botulinum toxin A (Botox Cosmetic): a review of its use in the treatment of glabellar frown lines. *Am J Clin Dermatol.* 2003;4(10):709–725.

CHAPTER

13

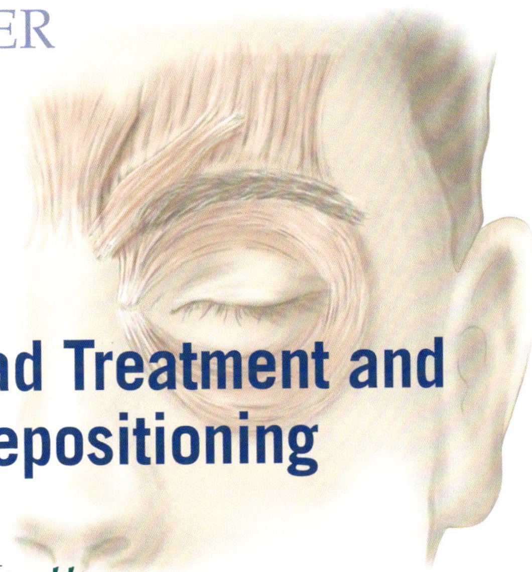

Forehead Treatment and Brow Repositioning

P. Daniel Knott

Treatment of the forehead and brows are intimately linked and are therefore best described together. Hyperkinetic lines of the forehead alone may be treated without affecting brow shape or position, and conversely brow contour and position may be adjusted without rejuvenating the forehead. However, treatment of one of these two areas usually influences the other, and treatment of one area must always be performed with attention directed to the other, in order to avoid untoward outcomes and displeased patients.

The position of the eyebrows is under constant adjustment by both the brow elevators and brow depressors. Brow position is a critical component of overall facial expressiveness and therefore caution should be exercised before adjusting the position with botulinum. This chapter introduces the major muscles involved in brow position, describes the simple and reliable methods of rejuvenating the forehead, and then discusses the finer points of brow reshaping.

ANATOMIC CONSIDERATIONS

The brows have been classically described as a having a club-shaped medial edge and a fine, tapered lateral border. Aesthetic ideals describe the medial and lateral borders having the same vertical height, with the peak located at a vertical tangent to the lateral aspect of the colored part of the eye (iris) or lateral canthus (Fig 13–1). The position of the medial border is controlled by the frontalis, the corrugator supercilli, the depressor supercilli, and the procerus. The position of the lateral tail is controlled by frontalis and the inferiorly oriented fibers of the orbicularis oculi.

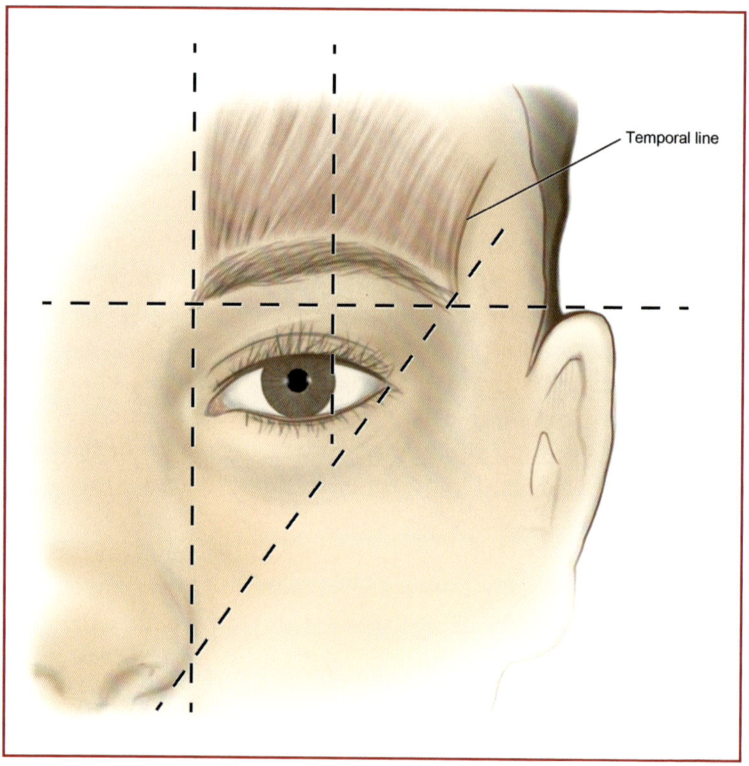

Figure 13–1

The orbicularis oculi is a very superficial muscle, located essentially directly below the dermis, and covered with a minimum of fat. The proximity of the orbicularis to the skin is what leads to the early development of "crow's feet" rhytids in many patients. The remaining muscles are usually covered by more extensive subcutaneous tissue.

ELEVATION VERSUS DEPRESSION

The frontalis muscle is the only brow elevator. Chemodenervation of this muscle with botulinum toxin therefore leads to effacement of the horizontally oriented rhytids and potential depression of the brow. As the brows usually become ptotic with age, caution must be exercised with patients in their fifth decade and beyond, when injecting this muscle in isolation, as it may result in a displeasing and unacceptably low brow. The remaining muscles mentioned above are brow depressors, and their chemodenervation may lead to subsequent brow elevation. Browplasty or brow elevation likewise will be more successful in younger patients due to their inherent muscle tone and connective tissue elasticity. Selective chemodenervation of different combinations of these muscles may lead to central brow elevation, tail elevation, relative medial club head depression, or complete elevation (Figure 13–2 shows the vectors of each of these muscles and relative strengths[1]).

INJECTION TECHNIQUE

Forehead

The horizontal rhytids in the forehead are caused by the contraction of the frontalis. This muscle may be continuous in the midline and extends from the supraorbital ridge to a superior

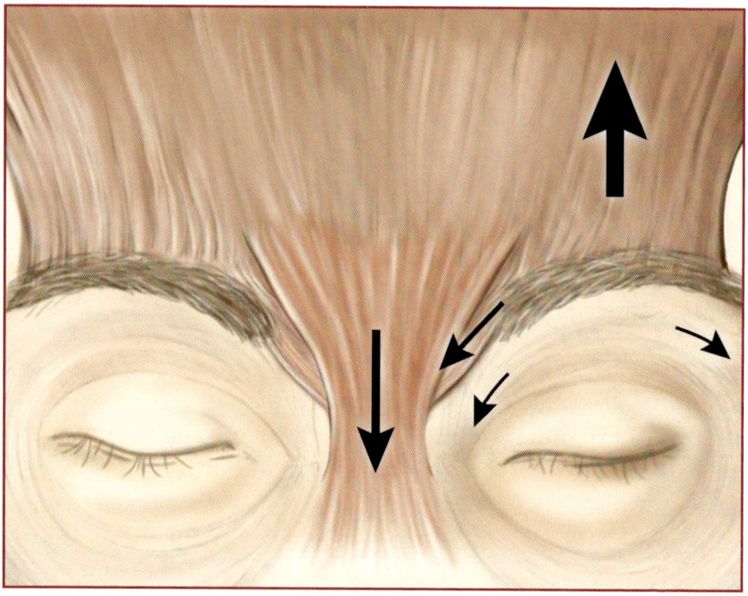

Figure 13–2

limit at or near the natural hairline. Its lateral border is defined by the temporal line, which is a curvilinear fascial confluence extending from the superolateral orbital rim near the lateral border of the brow up to the natural temporal hairline (see Fig 13–1). The temporal line separates the temple, containing the temporalis muscle, from the forehead, and injections targeting the forehead and brows need not be made lateral to this line.

During the office evaluation, a patient interested in brow rejuvenation should be asked to raise his or her eyebrows and the pattern of rhytids should be studied:

1. Do the rhytids cross the midline or is there a central area without wrinkles?
2. How strong are the contractions, and how close are they to the frontal hairline?
3. How much do the lateral brows elevate?

4. Are the rhytids present in repose or do they only manifest themselves with contraction?

If the wrinkles do not cross the midline, there is no need for central injections. Stronger contractions necessitate an increased dose of botulinum and rhytids at or near the hairline mandate injections performed higher on the forehead. If the lateral brows are not hyperactive, then I usually inject the forehead in an intramuscular plane in 4 to 6 points using 2 to 3 units of Botox Cosmetic (4 to 6 units of Dysport), with my lateral injections located approximately 2 cm above the lateral brow to preserve some muscle tone of the frontalis below this point, in order to preserve the positive emotive potential of the brows, while maintaining balance (**Fig 13–3**). If the lower, lateral frontalis is treated, the brow tails may depress, creating a sad expression. If a more dilute solution is chosen, then the unit dose may be reduced by 25 to 50%, usually without sacrificing effectiveness. If the rhytids are present in repose, then relatively higher doses are required in order to achieve maximal rhytid effacement. Patients with wrinkles only with frontalis contraction may benefit from prophylactic botulinum treatment, and therefore relatively lower doses are usually indicated. Younger patients with hyperkinetic forehead lines should be approached with caution, as they may be overusing their frontalis muscle to compensate for congenitally ptotic brows. Botulinum treatment of these individuals may lead to significant brow depression.[2]

Brow Reshaping

When brow elevation or reshaping is desired, botulinum toxin may be selectively used. Patients in their fifties and older usually experience minimal brow elevation with botulinum treatment, but among younger patients, 3 to 5 mm of lateral brow elevation may be achieved.[1] If the entire brow is to be raised,

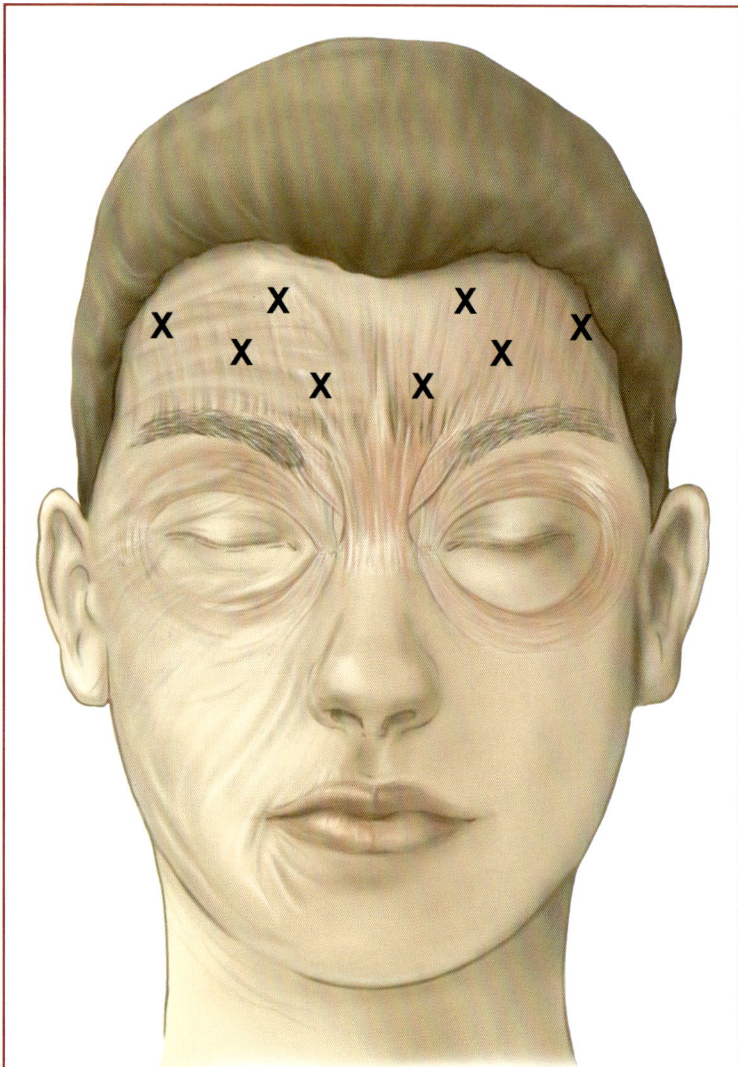

Figure 13–3

a selective corrugator and superolateral orbicularis injection is performed. The orbicularis is injected at the superior orbital rim in 2 doses of 2 to 3 units of Botulinum Cosmetic (4 to 6 units of Dysport) starting lateral to the mid-pupillary line (Fig 13–4). If the injection is made below the orbital rim, lid ptosis (blepharoptosis) may result.

If lateral brow ptosis is the primary complaint, then the brows may be rebalanced with botulinum toxin bringing about elevation of the brow tail and depression of the medial head.

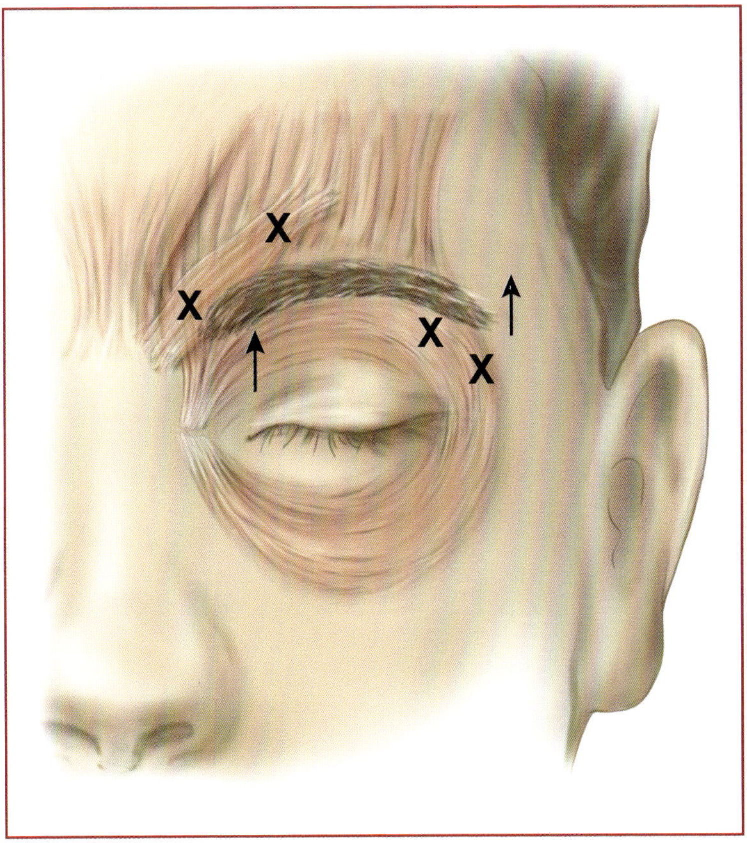

Figure 13–4

Frontalis injections are performed as above, preserving the lower lateral frontalis function between the midpupillary line and the temporal line. The corrugator or depressor supercilii muscles are not injected, in order to depress the medial brow, whereas the lateral tail will rise when crow's feet injections are performed as well (Fig 13–5). If this is inadequate, then additional injections along the descending fibers of the orbicularis lateral to the midpupillary line will further raise the tail (Fig 13–6). This should be done selectively otherwise the entire lateral tail will flare, creating a very unnatural expression.[3] Usually this technique is most effective among patients in their third to fifth decades of life.

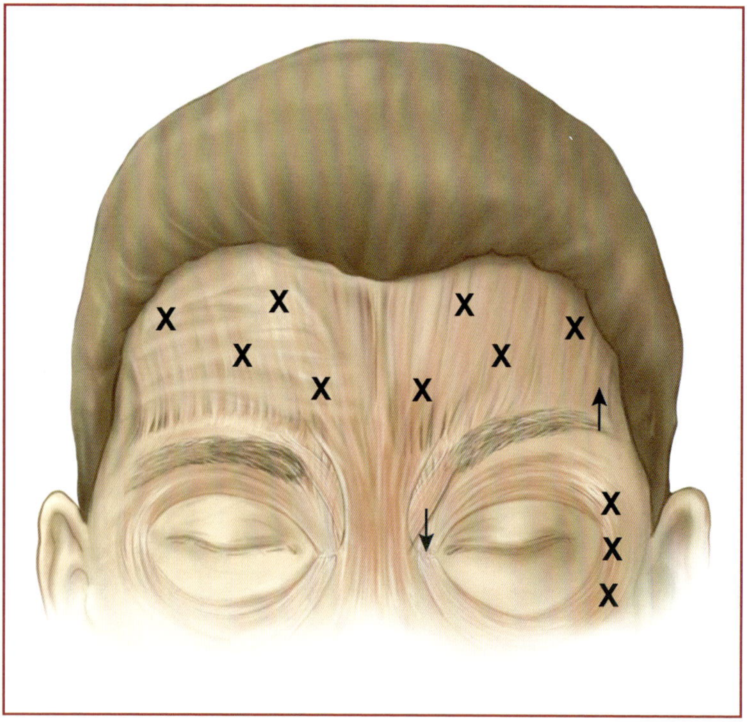

Figure 13–5

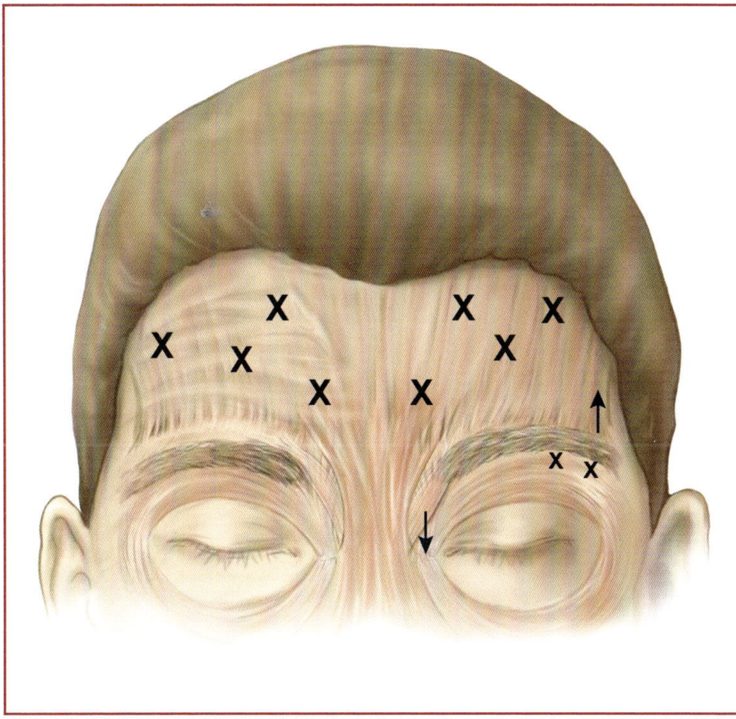

Figure 13–6

REFERENCES

1. Maas CS, Kim EJ. Temporal brow lift using botulinum toxin A: an update. *Plast Reconstr Surg.* 2003;112:109S–112S.
2. Rzany B, Dill-Muller D, Grablowitz D, et al. Repeated botulinum toxin A injections for the treatment of lines in the upper face: a retrospective study of 4103 treatments in 945 patients. *Dermatol Surg.* 2007;33:S18–25.
3. Salti G, Ghersetich I. Advanced botulinum toxin techniques against wrinkles in the upper face. *Clin Dermatol.* 2008;26:182–191.

CHAPTER

14

Periorbital Rejuvenation

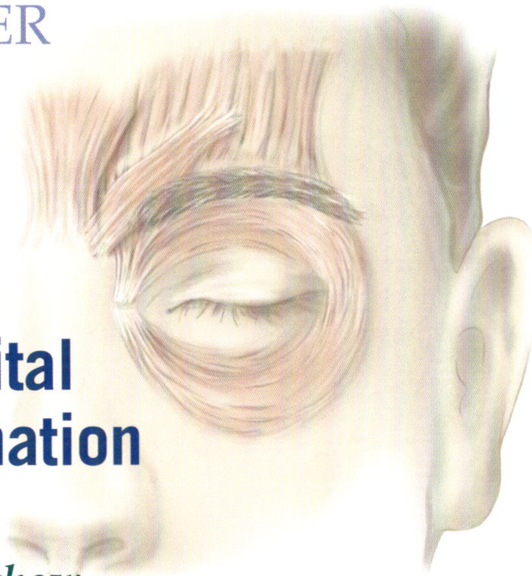

Andrea Jarchow

Age-related changes in the soft tissues around the eyes contribute to a fatigued appearance. A youthful look relies on smooth contours at the lateral and inferior orbital rim. Although certain surgical approaches may mitigate this appearance, the intermittent use of botulinum toxin is a less invasive avenue to a youthful appearance. An understanding of the muscular anatomy of the periorbital region is important in achieving a desired cosmetic outcome while avoiding complications. Botulinum toxin is a powerful tool and inadvertent uses may lead to unpleasant or unsightly cosmesis. Haphazard injections within the periorbital region may develop into severe functional deficits. Depth of injections as well as placement of injections are emphasized in this chapter.

ANATOMIC CONSIDERATIONS

The orbicularis oculi can be divided into 3 portions: pretarsal, preseptal, and orbital (Fig 14–1). The muscles' vector of contraction is primarily horizontal, tightening the upper and lower lids and bringing their free edges together. This chapter focuses on treatment of the lower lid and lateral orbital regions. The pretarsal region, overlying the tarsal plate, contributes mini-

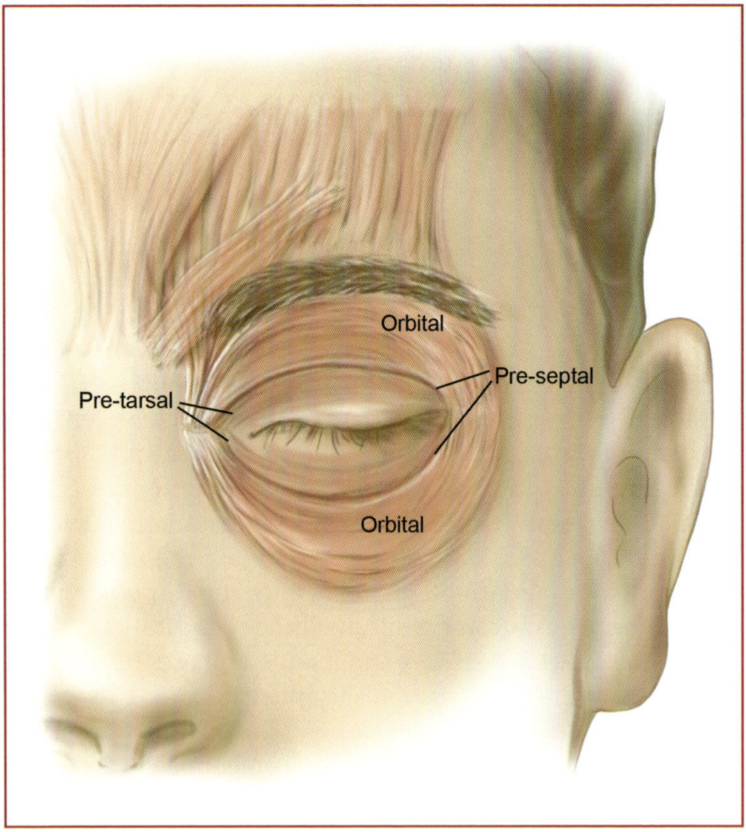

Figure 14–1

mally to periorbital rhytids. It assists in involuntary eye closure.[1] Injection of the pretarsal musculature with botulinum toxin is not common and is not recommended.

The preseptal and orbital portions of the muscle may hypertrophy and contribute to lower eyelid lines. Contraction allows for light eye closure as well as assists with blinking. Small quantities of botulinum may be injected into this muscle in the lower lid. A snap test and distraction test is recommended prior to injection in order to assess inherent lower lid orbicularis tone. If either of these tests demonstrates excess laxity, botulinum injections are not recommended, as chemical induced lower lid ectropion (eversion of the eyelid) and/or epiphora (tears accumulating in the lower eyelid trough and running down the cheeks) may result.

Repeated contraction of the orbital segment of the orbicularis oculi in combination with loss of collagen in the dermis and thinning of the skin give rise to the lateral orbital rhytids better known as crow's feet, which extend beyond the bony orbit and may involve the temple and upper cheek. These periorbital hyperdynamic lines may also extend medially under the lower eyelid and approach the medial canthus.

INJECTION TECHNIQUE

Patient consultation for periorbital injection begins with a thorough medical history. Particular attention should be given to the patient's ocular history (for example: thyroid eye disease, dry eye syndrome, previous surgery, etc). Inquiry into prior periorbital injection history may provide information into previous success and failure.

Injections are usually initiated in the lateral orbital segment of the orbicularis oculi using 2 to 4 injection sites with total dosing per orbit ranging from 8 to 12 units of Botox Cosmetic (16 to 32 units of Dysport).[2] The patient is asked to smile to demonstrate the distribution of the crow's feet. Injections are placed on or lateral to the bony lateral orbital rim approximately 0.5 cm apart (Fig 14–2). The injections are placed within the dermis due to the thin and superficial nature of the orbicularis oculi, avoiding the sensitive periosteum just deep to the muscle. A superficial injection is also less likely to cause bruising. A threading technique using a single, long needle pass may also be used, but is rarely indicated.

Caution: Placing the injection too close to the orbit or injecting too deep can lead to epiphora, lagophthalmos, and diplopia.

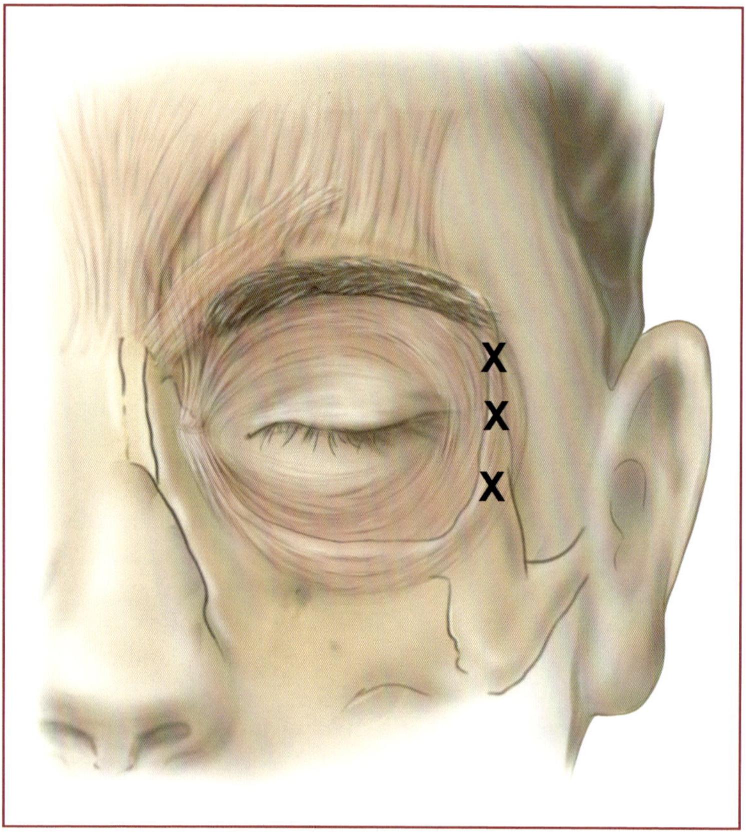

Figure 14–2

Placing the injection too deep over the malar eminence can lead to upper lip ptosis. More common complications include pain, bruising, and mild erythema at the injection sites.[3,4]

For patients with noted inferior eyelid lines or hypertrophy of the orbicularis, 2 to 4 units of Botox Cosmetic (4 to 8 units of Dysport) can be placed medially on or immediately below the inferior orbital rim (Fig 14–3). Using a new 30-gauge needle, 1 to 2 injections are given near the midpupillary line approximately 3 mm inferior to the eyelashes. In addition, to

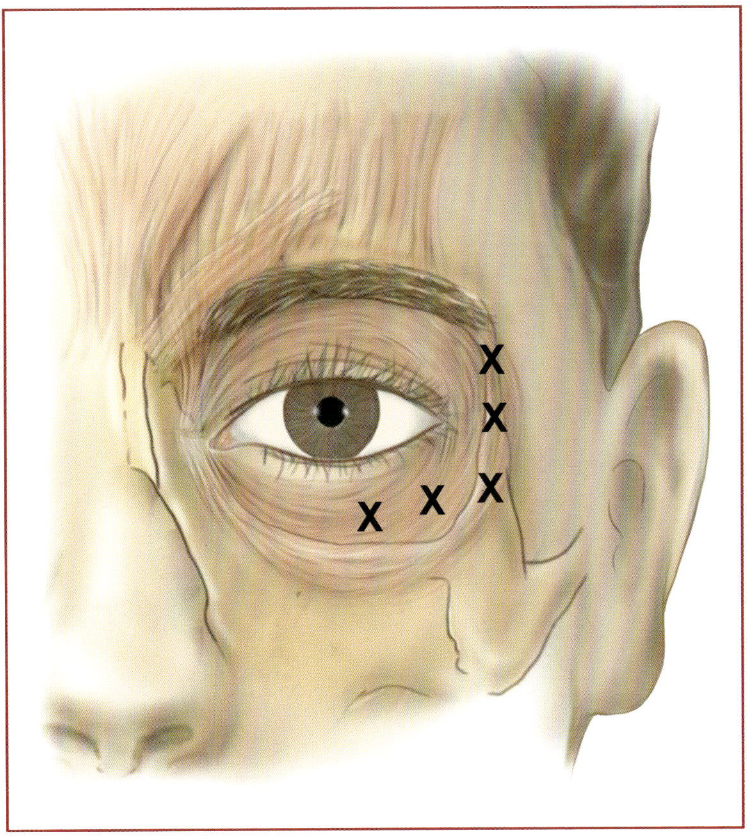

Figure 14–3

a softened appearance, patients may also note an increase in the vertical aperture opening, resulting in a more awake and alert look.

Caution: This injection, however, is not commonly performed due to the concern for iatrogenic ectropion and/or epiphora. Any concern about excess laxity should preclude injection. Furthermore, injections should not be made medial to the midpupillary line, as this may lead to epiphora.

REFERENCES

1. Zide BM. Anatomy of the eyelids. *Clin Plast Surg.* Oct. 1981; 8(4): 623–634.
2. Flynn TC, Carruthers JA, Carruthers A, et al. Botulinum A toxin (Botox) in the lower eyelid: dose-finding study. *Dermatol Surg.* Sept. 2003; 29(9): 943–950.
3. Matarasso SL, Matarasso A. Treatment guidelines for botulinum toxin type A for the periocular region and a report on partial upper lip ptosis following injections to the lateral canthal rhytids. *Plast Reconstr Surg.* July 2001; 108(1): 208–214.
4. Matarasso A, Deva AK, and the American Society of Plastic Surgeons DATA Committee. Botulinum toxin: safety and efficacy report. *Plast Reconstr Surg.* March 2002; 109(3): 1191–1197.

CHAPTER

15

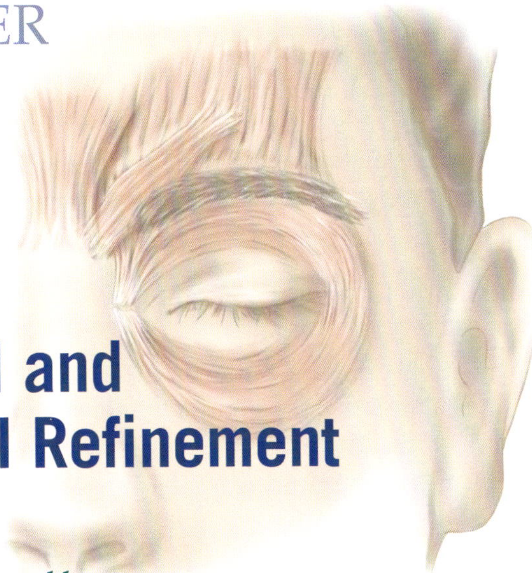

Perioral and Cervical Refinement

P. Daniel Knott

Although neuroparalytics are most effective when used in the upper third of the face, careful and selective use may also be applicable in the perioral region. The perioral region is divided into lip elevators, the oral sphincter, and the lip depressors. Although treatment of the oral sphincter (orbicularis oris) is the most common, all of these areas may benefit from appropriate treatment with botulinum toxin.

ANATOMIC CONSIDERATIONS AND INJECTION TECHNIQUE

Lip Elevators

The lip elevators include the levator anguli oris, the levator anguli superiorus alaeque nasi, zygomaticus major, and the zygomaticus minor. Each of these contribute to the formation of the nasolabial crease. Although not commonly performed, treatment of the lip elevators is possible when treating hyperfunctional smiles (gummy smiles). Treatment consists of 2 to 3 units of Botox Cosmetic (4 to 6 units of Dysport) per side immediately inferior and lateral to the lateral ala (Fig 15–1). Successful treatment will lower the lip during full smiling, and reduce gingival show.[1]

Orbicularis Oris (Oral sphincter)

As mentioned in the section on theory of aesthetic use of botulinum toxin, repetitive contraction and relaxation of the orbicularis oris sphincter around the mouth during speaking and swallowing/eating leads to the progressive development of "smoker's lines" oriented around the mouth, much like spokes emanating from a bicycle axle. The natural creases are evident during puckering, as the skin is bunched up above the contracting muscle. With persistent use, the rhytids begin to form,

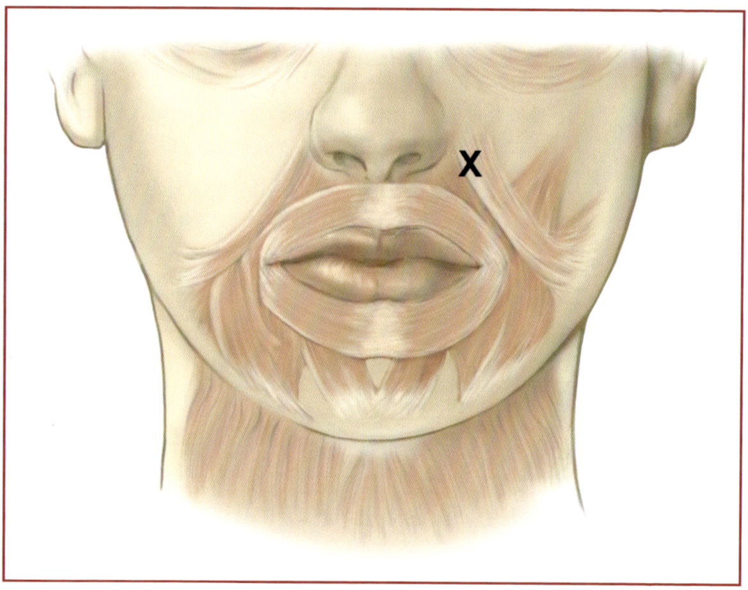

Figure 15–1

usually in the 4th decade of life, and eventually deepen as the skin looses its natural elasticity through aging and solar exposure, and the overlying soft tissue atrophies. These rhytids are superficial and fine, and may be treated with superficial peeling/laser treatments. However, there are commonly several deeper rhytids, with at least one located in each of the four quadrants around the lips. These deeper lines may be successfully treated with botulinum toxin.

The orbicularis oris is a powerful muscle, which is located a medium depth beneath the skin. Botulinum should be injected directly into the middle of the rhytid, near the vermilion border, and 1 to 2 units of Botox Cosmetic (2–4 units of Dysport) may be used initially (Fig 15–2). The cupid's bow and oral commissures should be avoided. Injection of more than 1 rhytid per perioral quadrant is not recommended, as overinjection may lead to noticeable adynamic areas, and severe overinjection may even lead to loss of oral competence.[2–5]

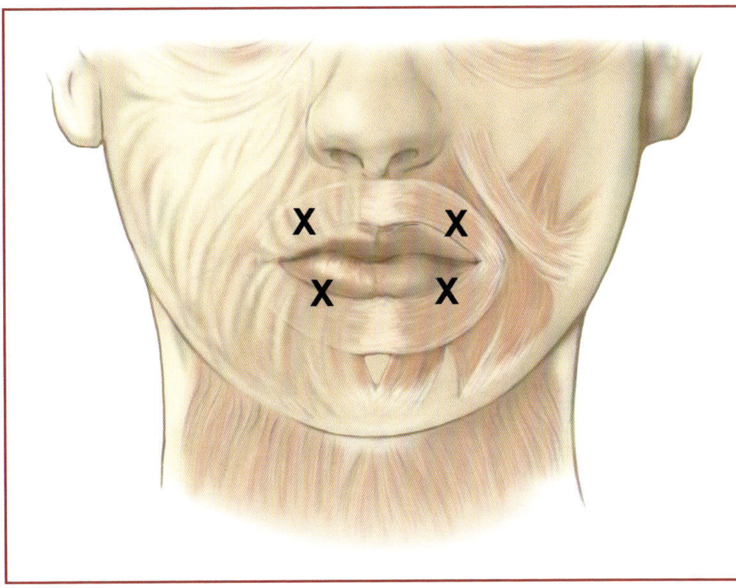

Figure 15–2

Lip Depressors

The mentalis, the depressor labii inferiorus, and the depressor anguli oris are the three lip depressors. Treatment of the paralyzed lower lip is reserved for the chapter on facial paralysis.

The depressor anguli oris arises from the oblique line of the mandible and inserts into the oral commissure. Repetitive contraction draws the commissure inferiorly and deepens the melomental folds. Three to 6 units of Botox Cosmetic (6–12 units of Dysport) may be injected deeply into the intramuscular plane on each side, midway between the oral commissure and the inferior aspect of the mandible, thereby softening the "marionette lines" and bringing the corners of the mouth upwards, creating a less aged expression (Fig 15–3).

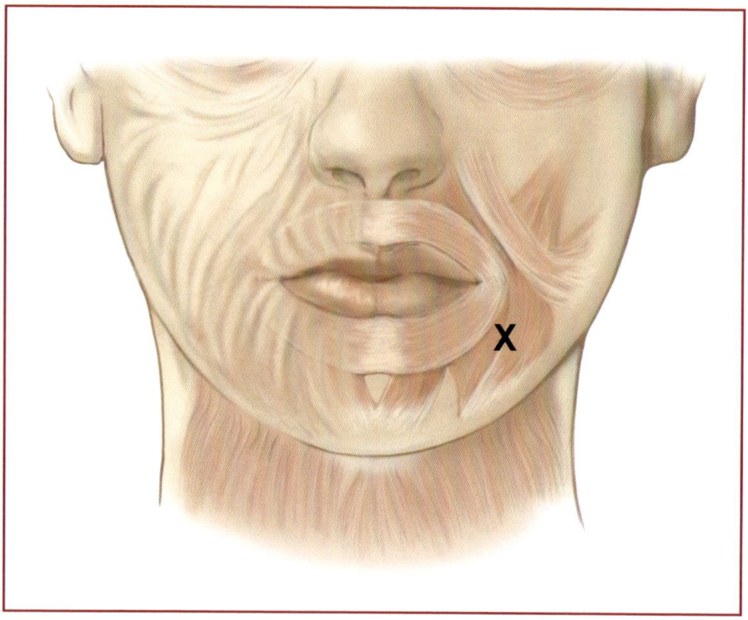

Figure 15–3

The mentalis muscle originates from the inferior aspect of the mandibular midline and inserts into the dermis above and below the mental crease. Contraction of this muscle propels the lip upward and outward, helping to create a pout. This muscle is also responsible for deepening the mental crease. For patients with an excessively deep crease, injection of botulinum toxin into the mentalis may provide effective treatment. Four to 6 units of Botox Cosmetic (8–12 units of Dysport) may be injected into the mentalis muscle midway between the bottom of the chin and the mental crease (Fig 15–4). Attention to bilateral injection is important. Likewise, patients with so-called peau d'orange (orange peel chin), with multiple small puckerings, may also benefit from injection of the mentalis slightly below the point illustrated in Figure 15–4.

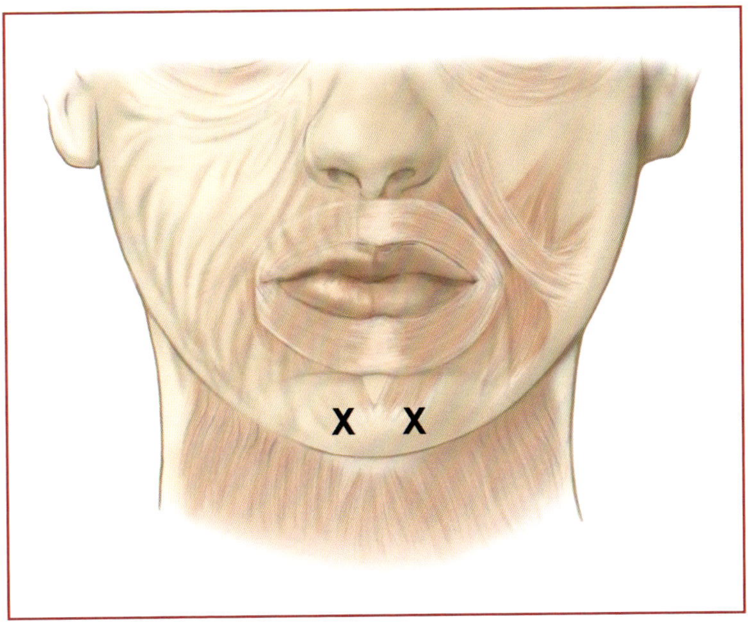

Figure 15–4

CERVICAL BANDS

Vertically oriented medial platysma bands are caused by age-related weakening of the fascia connecting the platysma in the midline. In very selected cases, when these bands are the most prominent component of the aging neck, and fat deposition, jowling, and significant skin excess are not present, botulinum toxin may play a role in rejuvenation.[7] Ten to 20 units of Botox Cosmetic (20–40 units of Dysport) may be injected intramuscularly 1 cm lateral to the bands in 1 or 2 subsites bilaterally, in order to soften the bands and harmonize the contour of the neck (Fig 15–5). Depending on the volume of cervical fat deposition, the platysma may be very superficial or quite deep. Therefore, in order to avoid inadvertent injection of deeper

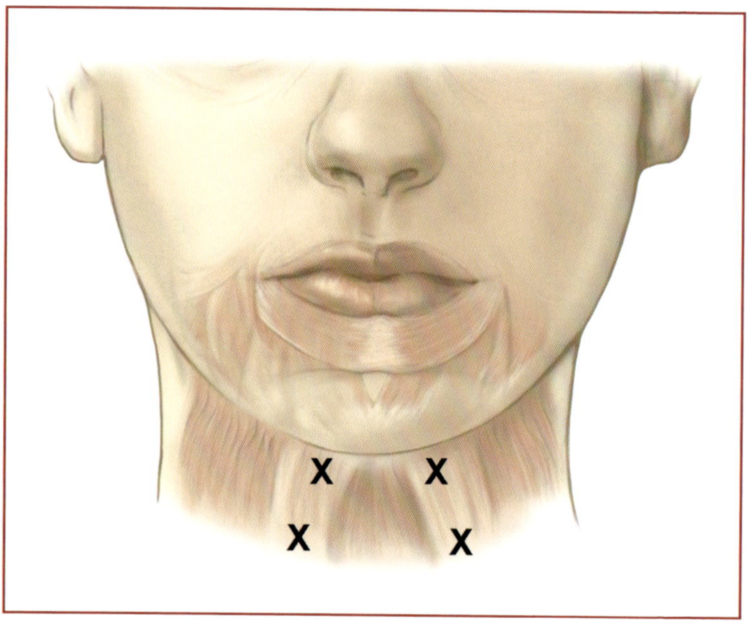

Figure 15–5

muscles important in mastication and swallowing, it is recommended to grasp the bands between the thumb and forefinger in order to correctly judge the depth of injection.

REFERENCES

1. Polo M. Botulinum toxin type A (botox) for the neuromuscular correction of excessive gingival display on smiling (gummy smile). *Am J Orthod Dentofacial Orthop*. 2008;133:195–203.
2. Perkins NW, Smith SP Jr, Williams EF 3rd. Perioral rejuvenation: complementary techniques and procedures. *Facial Plast Surg Clin North Am*. 2007:15:423–432.
3. Kane MA. The functional anatomy of the lower face as it applies to rejuvenation via chemodenervation. *Facial Plast Surg*. 2005;21:55–64.
4. Perkins SW, Sandel HDT. Anatomic considerations, analysis, and the aging process of the perioral region. *Facial Plast Surg Clin North Am*. 2007;15:403–407.
5. Kaplan Se, Sherris DA, Gassner HG, Friedman O. The use of botulinum toxin A in perioral rejuvenation. *Facial Plast Surg Clin North Am*. 2007;15:415–421.
6. Carruthers J, Carruthers A. Aesthetic botulinum A toxin in the mid and lower face and neck. *Dermatol Surg*. 2003;29:468–476.
7. Suryadevara, A. Update on perioral cosmetic enhancement. *Curr Opin Otolaryngol Head Neck Surg*. 2008;16:347–351.

CHAPTER

16

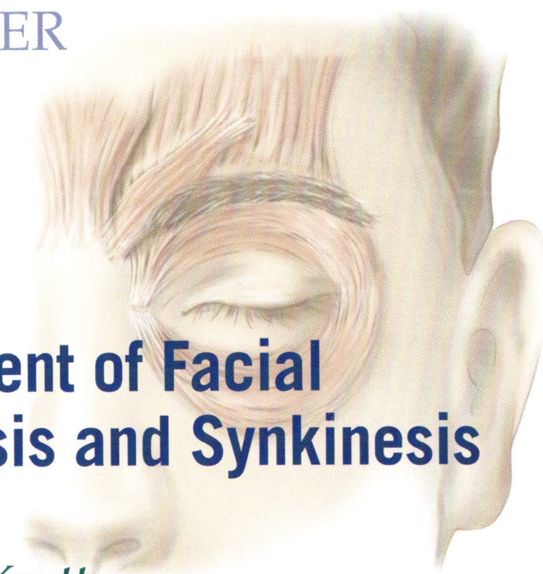

Treatment of Facial Paralysis and Synkinesis

P. Daniel Knott

The inability to manipulate the muscles of facial expression, as with facial paralysis, has profound communicative and social consequences. Whatever the etiology (cerebrovascular accident, CNS tumor, trauma, congenital, postsurgical, or idiopathic), patients with facial paralysis often shun human interaction and may frequently suffer from depression.[1,2]

Opportunities for facial reanimation are time dependent. In the setting of a permanent, complete paralysis, motor endplate degradation occurs within 1 to 2 years, and thereafter only static reanimation options are available to patients, with the exception of local and distant muscle transfers.[3] Synkinesis, the simultaneous contraction of some or all of the muscle groups supplied by facial nerve, may also follow partial or imperfect re-innervation, and is treated separately below.

Botulinum toxin is a powerful, yet simple adjunct to a comprehensive overall strategy for treating facial paralysis, and every approach to the treatment of patients with facial paralysis should include consideration of neuroparalytic therapy. Botulinum toxin may be used irrespective of time from onset of the paralysis, and therefore has a role in the treatment of temporary to permanent cases. The reversibility of botulinum permits its use in early, potentially temporary facial paralysis. Its limited duration of action requires re-dosing in cases of long-term or permanent paralysis.

When treating short-term or long-term facial paralysis (not synkinesis), subsites for injection are all located on the normal, nonparalyzed hemiface. This strategy is effective, as treatment attempts to restore symmetry at rest and in motion. The paralyzed side demonstrates muscle atrophy and loss/atrophy of rhytids. Therefore, balancing occurs through the softening or effacement of rhytids on the functioning facial half to restore symmetry at rest, and through selective chemodenervation to improve symmetry during animation.[4]

ANATOMIC CONSIDERATIONS AND INJECTION TECHNIQUE FOR FACIAL PARALYSIS

Upper Third of the Face (Forehead and Eyes)

Facial paralysis manifests in the upper third of the nonparalyzed hemiface with horizontal wrinkles and usual compensatory brow hyperfunction. Asymmetry is therefore present at rest and with animation. Symmetry is gained by treating the hyperfunctional frontalis with 8 to 12 units of Botox Cosmetic (16 to 24 units of Dysport) (Fig 16–1). This will improve the rhytid asymmetry and will depress the hyperfunctional brow, yielding balance at rest and with animation. This is the most straightforward and effective subsite for injection. Treatment of the periorbital complex may be limited to the lateral orbicularis oculi, responsible for the crow's feet wrinkles, in order to efface the rhytids and realize symmetry with the paralyzed side.

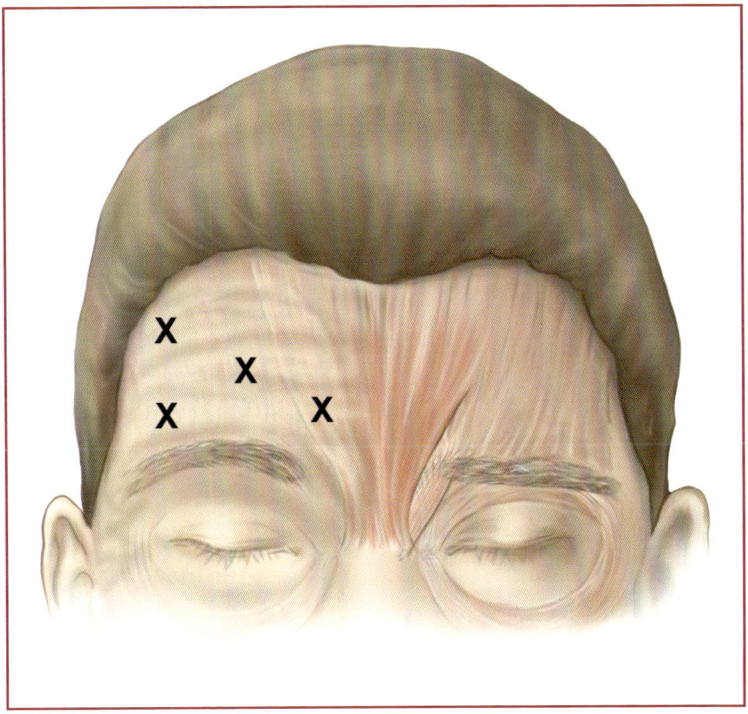

Figure 16–1

The approach should follow that as indicated in Chapter 14, and should never involve the preseptal or pretarsal orbicularis oculi (see Fig 14–2).

Middle Third (Cheeks and Upper Lips)

Treatment of the middle third of the face must be performed with caution and only after effective treatment of the upper third of the face has been achieved. Weakening the lip elevators on the functional side should be undertaken with caution in order to avoid impairing oral competence. Furthermore, any treatment to the extrinsic and intrinsic muscles of the nose may only exacerbate nasal valve collapse and nasal airway compromise that is commonly encountered on the paralyzed side. The orbicularis oris should not be injected. The zygomaticus major and the levator anguli oris may both be weakened by limited doses of toxin injected deeply into the intramuscular plane.[5]

The zygomaticus major originates in the subzygomatic fossa and inserts into the modiolus, adjacent to the oral commissure. The origin of the zygomaticus major may be palpated in the subzygomatic fossa, which is located posterior and inferior to the malar eminence and anterior to the zygomaticotemporal suture.[6] The zygomaticus major may be treated with no more than 2 injections of 4 units of Botox Cosmetic (8 units of Dysport). The first injection should be made near the fossa and the second may be made midway between the oral commissure and the subzygomatic fossa (Fig 16–2).

The levator anguli oris originates from the canine fossa, immediately below the infraorbital foramen. The infraorbital foramen may be palpated as a depression in the face of the maxilla inferior to the infraorbital rim directly below the midpupillary line. The levator anguli oris may be injected once with 4 units of Botox Cosmetic (8 units of Dysport) directly below the infraorbital foramen (see Fig 16–2). If treated, the injection should be directed to its origin to minimize the potential for diffusion to the orbicularis oris muscle fibers.

Lower Third (Lower Lips and Chin)

Similar to the middle third of the face, treatment of the lower third should not impair oral competence. Therefore, caution should be used to avoid weakening the orbicularis oris. Asymmetry is caused primarily by dysfunction of the lower lip depressors (depressor labii inferioris, and depressor anguli oris). Depressor function is usually hyperactive, taking part in the compensatory hyperfunction of the nonparalyzed hemiface.

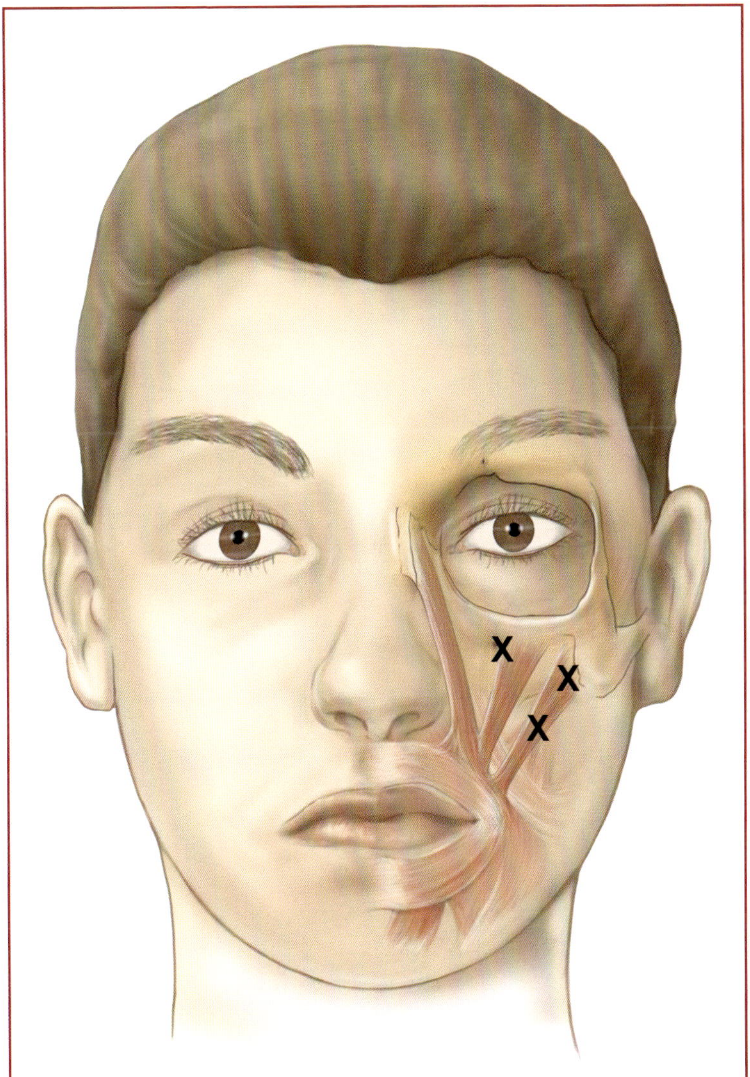

Figure 16–2

The depressor anguli oris arises from the anteroinferior border of the mandible (oblique line) on a line drawn directly inferior and slightly lateral to the oral commissure and inserts into the modiolus. Five units of Botox Cosmetic (10 units of Dysport) may be injected at medium depth midway between the oral commissure and the inferior border of the mandible (Fig 16–3).

The depressor labii inferioris also arises from the antero-inferior border of the mandible (oblique line) on a line drawn directly inferior and slightly medial to the oral commissure and inserts into the lower lip medial to the commissure after blending with the fibers of the orbicularis oris. Five units of Botox Cosmetic (10 units of Dysport) may therefore be injected midway between the inferior border of the mandible and the lower lip vermilion border, slightly medial to the vertical tangent to the oral commissure (see Fig 16–3). This point should be 1 to 2 cm medial to the point of injection used to treat the depressor anguli oris.

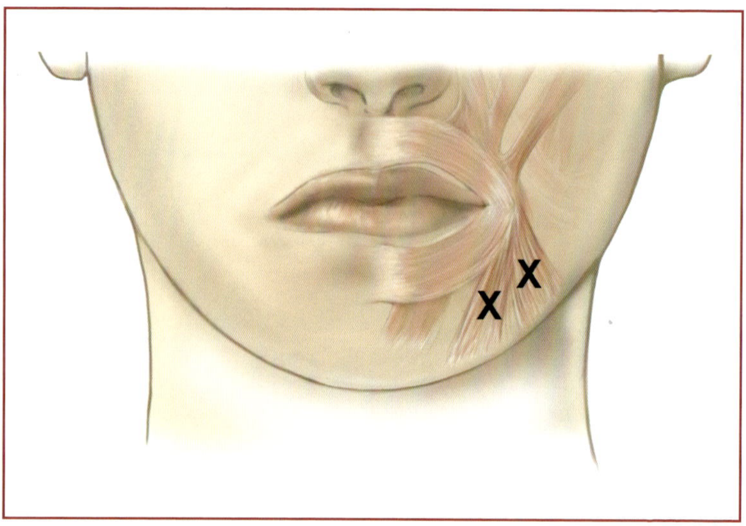

Figure 16–3

SYNKINESIS

This is among the most common of facial paralytic complaints. Synkinesis means simultaneous movement and usually affects patients following cerebrovascular accidents, idiopathic facial paralysis (Bell's palsy), herpes zoster oticus, or trauma. Synkinesis may involve any or all of the muscles of facial expression over the affected hemiface and manifests with involuntary facial muscle movement accompanying a voluntary movement. Synkinesis is the ultimate aberrant recovery phase of a partial or total facial paralysis, and occurs in a nonvolitional manner. The dominant patterns of synkinesis are the mouth corner synkinesis coupled to voluntary brow lift and/or eye closure movements and synkineses of the eye coupled to voluntary movement lip puckering or smiling.[7]

In contrast to the section above covering facial paralysis, neuroparalytic treatment of synkinesis is directed to the once-paralyzed side, that is, the side exhibiting synkinetic movement. However, as detailed below, many patients benefit from bilateral treatment as well as facial movement re-education therapy.[8]

ANATOMIC CONSIDERATIONS AND INJECTION TECHNIQUE FOR SYNKINESIS

Prioritization must occur, with preservation of oral competence and prevention of exposure keratitis. Successful treatment of synkinesis with botulinum toxin causes selective, partial facial paralysis and therefore results in asymmetry. Therefore, optimal rebalancing occurs when certain muscles are treated on both the synkinetic and normal sides, in order to preserve symmetry. The lower lip depressors (depressor anguli oris and depressor labii inferioris) and frontalis muscles all may be treated bilaterally following the instructions above, but this is rarely indicated. As mentioned, usually the synkinetic movement is limited to involuntary upper lip elevation and involuntary eye closure. Treatment of the upper lip elevators should target the muscle most responsible for the synkinetic movement, and this needs to be determined through careful patient observation. Botulinum toxin treatment should be directed to this muscle (usually the zygomaticus major or minor and/or orbicularis oris). Treatment of the zygomaticus may follow that detailed in Figure 16–2, and treatment of the orbicularis oris should be conservative using doses of botulinum as detailed in Figure 15–2 in Chapter 15.

Treatment of a synkinetic orbicularis oculi is much more complicated. Neuroparalytic intervention should be undertaken only in conjunction with a strategy designed to avoid exposure keratitis that could follow the development of lagophthalmos resulting from a paralyzed orbicularis oculi. A multidisciplinary approach incorporating the skills and experience of an oculoplastic, facial plastic, or general plastic surgeon is recommended, usually involving the placement of weights (gold or platinum) in the upper lid and lower lid tightening procedures. In this setting, the upper lid and infrabrow complex should be treated with 2 to 3 superficial injections of 2 to 3 units of Botox Cosmetic (4–6 units of Dysport) (Fig 16–4).

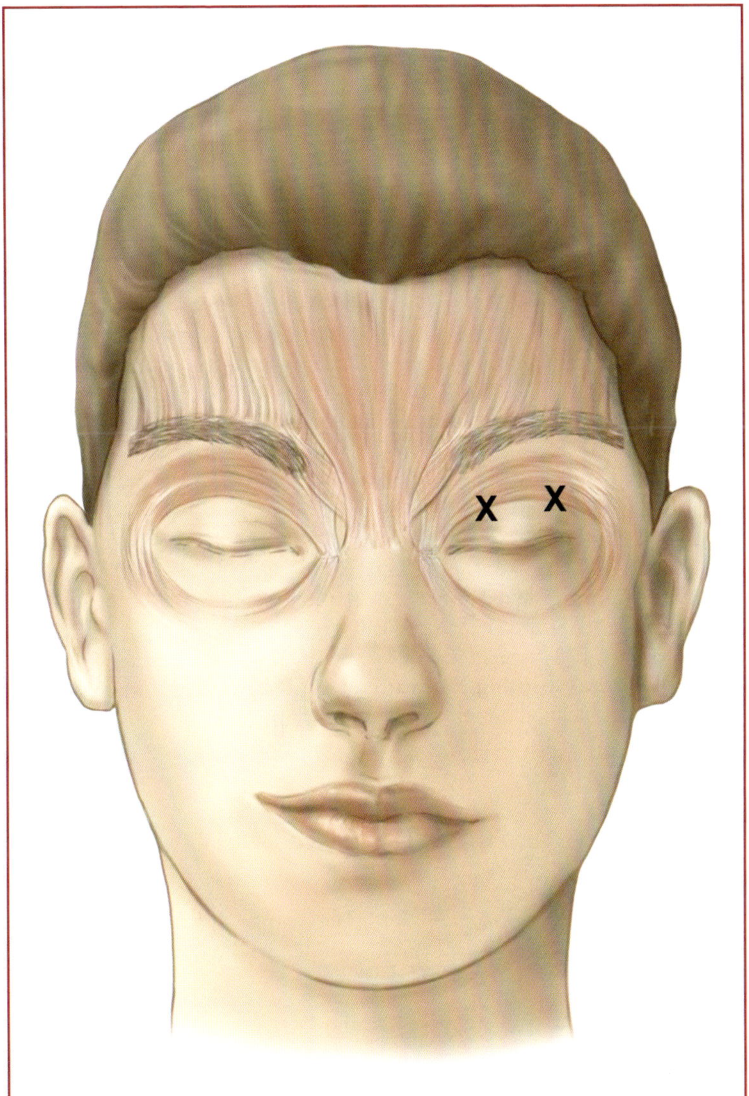

Figure 16–4

REFERENCES

1. Ryzenman JM, Pensak ML, Tew JM Jr. Facial paralysis and surgical rehabilitation: a quality of life analysis in a cohort of 1,595 patients after acoustic neuroma surgery. *Otol Neurotol.* 2005;26(3):516–521.
2. Tate JR, Tollefson TT. Advances in facial reanimation. *Curr Opin Otolaryngol Head Neck Surg.* 2006;14(4):242–248.
3. Myckatyn TM, Mackinnon SE. The surgical management of facial nerve injury. *Clin Plas Surg.* 2003;30(2):307–318.
4. Salles AG, Toledo PN, Ferreira MC. Botulinum toxin injection in long-standing facial paralysis patients: improvement of facial symmetry observed up to 6 months. *Aesth Plast Surg.* 2009;33:582–590.
5. Bikhazi NB, Maas CS. Refinement in the rehabilitation of the paralyzed face using botulinum toxin. *Otolaryngol Head Neck Surg.* 1997; 117:303–307.
6. Miller PJ, Smith S, Shah A. The subzygomatic fossa: a practical landmark in identifying the zygomaticus major muscle. *Arch Facial Plast Surg.* 2007;9(4):271–274.
7. Beurskens CH, Oosterhof J, Nijhuis-van der Sanden MW. Frequency and location of synkineses in patients with peripheral facial nerve paresis. *Otol Neurotol.* 2010;31(4):671–675.
8. Borodic GE, Cheney M, McKenna M. Contralateral injections of botulinum A toxin for the treatment of hemifacial spasm to achieve increased facial symmetry. *Plast Reconstr Surg.* 1992;90:972–977.

Index

A

B

C

D

E

F

G